RESEARCH LITERACY
for HEALTH and COMMUNITY PRACTICE

Sonya L. Jakubec and
Barbara J. Astle

RESEARCH LITERACY
for HEALTH and COMMUNITY PRACTICE

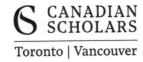
CANADIAN
SCHOLARS
Toronto | Vancouver

Research Literacy for Health and Community Practice
By Sonya L. Jakubec and Barbara J. Astle

First published in 2017 by
Canadian Scholars
425 Adelaide Street West, Suite 200
Toronto, Ontario
M5V 3C1

www.canadianscholars.ca

Library and Archives Canada Cataloguing in Publication

Jakubec, Sonya L., author

Research literacy for health and community practice / Sonya L. Jakubec and Barbara J. Astle.

Includes bibliographical references and index.
Issued in print and electronic formats.
ISBN 978-1-55130-991-0 (softcover).--ISBN 978-1-55130-993-4
(EPUB).--ISBN 978-1-55130-992-7 (PDF)

    1. Nursing--Research--Textbooks. 2. Textbooks. I. Astle, Barbara J., 1957-, author II. Title.

RT81.5.J35 2017   610.73072   C2017-902609-7   C2017-902610-0

Cover design by Elisabeth Springate
Interior design by Brad Horning

17   18   19   20   21   5   4   3   2   1

Printed and bound in Canada by Webcom

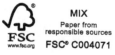

MIX
Paper from
responsible sources
FSC® C004071

CONTENTS

Chapter 9

LIST OF FIGURES, TABLES, AND BOXES

Figures

Tables

Boxes

PREFACE

In a world where knowledge is expanding exponentially and more easily accessed than ever before, it is essential that students and practitioners in fields of health and community service are able to clearly understand and communicate basic research concepts. The quality and safety of contemporary health and community practice depend, in part, on this literacy.

This introductory textbook is appropriate for undergraduate students involved in (inter)professional practices in health, community services, and other fields. It offers readers an opportunity to increase their understanding of the process of engaging with research literature and other studies at a beginning level. *Research Literacy for Health and Community Practice* is written in a style that makes understanding basic research concepts less intimidating and more user-friendly. This textbook offers a wealth of critical thinking exercises, recommended readings, online resources, and practical in-class activities to apply and engage readers in the basic research literacy concepts presented.

It was our intention that this first edition of *Research Literacy for Health and Community Practice* help beginning undergraduate students to understand the importance of research literacy as an essential competency for evidence-informed practice in health and community practice disciplines. As well, we have been intentional about highlighting the distinction between *research literacy*, as the acquiring of skills to find, understand, and critically evaluate evidence to apply to their practice, and *research capacity*, as the acquiring of skills to conduct research. This is not a research methods text, instructing on the research process involved in *conducting* a research study; rather, it guides users with a basic understanding of what it means to be *research literate*, and to draw upon this literacy in interprofessional practice settings.

The book is organized into chapters that build toward a basic comprehension and conversational ability with the language of research for evidence-informed practice. Concepts related to information, research, evidence for practice, and knowledge and evidence in practice are introduced at a basic level, with examples and exercises to gain comfort with the more technical language. Distinct chapters about searching the literature and critical appraisal of different approaches to research are central to building understanding and conversational skills in research. While distinct, these chapters build toward a growing literacy and are intended to be read in order. Learning objectives are provided at the start of each chapter. Examples and key information are highlighted in text boxes; and relevant and numerous learning activities and practice exam questions are provided in the appendices. Concepts are defined in more depth in the glossary toward the end of the book. As with any language- and literacy-focused book, the glossary is a resource to be used throughout the learning experience. Additional instructor resources are also available to accompany this book.

We remind students that literacy is an evolving process, something that will develop through reading, contributing to informed and open-minded discussions, participating in research studies, taking advanced research courses, acting as assistants in research work, and simply learning about the process through experience. Just as with learning a new language, students must begin with the basics of the process and structures of the culture and language of research, have a foundational vocabulary, immerse in a variety of different aspects of the language, practise (as with the learning activities appended to each chapter), make some mistakes, and have some fun!

ACKNOWLEDGEMENTS

Writing a book encompasses the collaboration of many people committed to the idea, dedicated time, numerous tasks, and then the achievement of such a goal. We would like to acknowledge and thank the superb editorial and production professionals at Canadian Scholars/Women's Press, the contributors, global reviewers, and our families, students, and colleagues.

Initially, the idea for this book transpired while we were teaching research courses to undergraduate nursing students at Mount Royal University, Calgary, Alberta, Canada. During this time, we pondered about how our students were learning and critically applying the concepts of research to inform their practice. As we developed our conceptual thinking and practical learning activities, we thought about writing a book to specifically address the concept of *research literacy* for our students in nursing, midwifery, and other community practice disciplines. We brought our initial ideas to Keriann McGoogan (Acquisitions Editor) who helped us bring our vision to Canadian Scholars/Women's Press. We are so grateful for her encouragement, support, and practical work of bridging the varying requirements of authors and the publisher in the early stages of the project. Natalie Garriga, Development Editor, Canadian Scholars/Women's Press, continued to provide exemplary professionalism and overall management of the project. We could not have completed this book without her ongoing support, direction, and patience. Cari Merkley, Academic Librarian and Associate Professor, brought her information literacy and health reference expertise as the contributing author for chapter 4. Cari's deep commitment and dedication to the teaching and learning of research provided us with a continual reminder of our purpose for this book. To the global reviewers who shared their expertise and knowledge about research, Shanaya Nelson, our meticulous copy editor, and the production professionals with Canadian Scholars/Women's Press, who assisted us in crafting a clear, literate, and practical book—we are deeply indebted to all of you. As well, throughout this process, our families, students, and colleagues continued to remind us that the effort was worth the inevitable sacrifices, and this book would not have been produced without all of your support! Ultimately, we must thank each other. Working in a writing and project partnership, such as this book, is like a long road trip with the exciting time of planning, sharing the driver's seat during some of the longer days, and finally reaching the destination—as good colleagues and friends, grateful to have taken the journey together!

Sonya L. Jakubec
Barbara J. Astle

1 | INTRODUCTION TO RESEARCH LITERACY FOR HEALTH AND COMMUNITY PRACTICE

> "Basically, I'm not interested in doing research ... I'm interested in understanding, which is quite a different thing."
>
> —David Blackwell

LEARNING OBJECTIVES

This chapter focuses on understanding how research literacy is relevant to health and community practice. We first present an overview to introduce the chapters included in this textbook, which is then followed by a description of how you can use this textbook in your practice. After reading this chapter and completing the practical learning activities in appendix B, you will be able to do the following:

- Describe research literacy as an issue related to health and community practice.
- Describe the definitions and history of research literacy for professional practitioners.
- Understand how to read and use this textbook.

CHAPTER OUTLINE

- An Introduction to Research Literacy
  - Definitions and History
- Objectives of the Text and Chapter Summaries
- Description of Ways to Approach and Use the Text
- Review and Reflect

AN INTRODUCTION TO RESEARCH LITERACY

The term *research literacy* does not describe just the ability to read research. There are consequences to misinformed and uncritical health and community practice, and research literacy is a key element of providing competent practice within and across these fields (Finch, 2007). As an example, parents may be misinformed and undecided on whether or not they wish to vaccinate their children; it is important that they are provided with substantive evidence to allow them to make an informed decision. The questions you should ask: What is suitable evidence for decision making in health and community practice? What constitutes "sufficient proof" or "good" evidence (Ciliska, Thomas, & Buffett, 2008)? Everyone has different answers to those questions. The matters of knowledge, evidence, and use of knowledge in practice are complex and can be highly political (Rycroft-Malone et al., 2004; Thomas, Burt, & Parkes, 2010).

To formulate a truly informed opinion on a subject, issue, or problem in health and community practice, you need to become familiar with both the ethical and political matters of knowledge making, and to be able to critically appraise current research in your field. To do that, you have to read *primary research literature* (often just called *the literature*) and a variety of other research papers. This task can seem overwhelming just because of the sheer volume of literature available. In addition, when it comes to reading a research paper, you may have experienced frustration due to the complex academic writing and the unfamiliar jargon; and perhaps you have read the abstract but skipped over the methods and results sections to read the conclusions without questioning the purpose, process, and approach used.

Understanding when reading research papers is an important skill to learn for those seeking an advanced professional degree in the health sciences, social sciences, and other related disciplines. You can learn it, but like any skill or new language, it takes patience, practice, and persistence. Throughout this textbook, we compare the development of this new skill to learning a new language. First, you learn the basic greetings and how to order from a menu, and then you learn the more in-depth techniques of grammar and structure within a language. The language of research is no different—first, you learn the basic principles, the foundations on which research is built, and then you learn the structure of it so you can read research papers critically and knowledgeably.

The intention of this textbook is to assist you to become more literate about research in order to approach reading and understanding research papers with greater ease and confidence. We also strive to help you acquire the skills to be able to access the world of research and converse in its language. *Research Literacy for Health and Community Practice* does not address what would be needed for new researchers to design and conduct their own research study (there are many excellent resources, training and educational courses, and workshops that can prepare beginning and more advanced researchers in their projects). Rather, this textbook provides an overview of knowledge making and the skills to search, read, and understand research papers. It will support you in learning how to conduct a literature review, critique research findings and conclusions, and understand how research may be used in your professional practice. This textbook is appropriate for students and interprofessional practitioners in health-related and social science disciplines who may have little background in sciences, community services, or health care. Professionals in practice disciplines such as nursing, midwifery, practical nursing, social work, and child and elder care, as well as those working in related health and community practices such as recreation therapy, massage therapy, respiratory therapy, and other fields need to develop research literacy, and this textbook is a place to begin. The textbook is based on the assumption that readers are interested in developing a *basic* understanding of a research paper and being able to decide whether or not it is a credible study that might have application in their practice.

The kind of scientific articles we explore are referred to as *primary research papers*. These are peer-reviewed reports of new research on a specific question (or questions). Another useful type of publication is a review paper. Review papers or *systematic reviews* are also peer-reviewed, but do not present new information; rather, they summarize multiple primary research articles to give a sense of the consensus, debates, and unanswered questions within a field. Critical appraisal of review articles is also necessary, considering that these reviews are only a snapshot of the research at the time they are published. For example, a review paper on studies about the management of pandemics (e.g., the "Hong Kong Flu" in 1968–1969) will provide foundational knowledge, but may not be as informative for practice when dealing with more recent pandemics (e.g., H1N1, also called the swine flu, in 2009), or informing practice in 2017 for the next pandemic. However, fields change considerably over time, as do the questions and concerns within the context and environment. Therefore, research literacy is an ongoing lifelong endeavour!

Professionals in health and community disciplines are required to continuously examine their own practice and develop their knowledge, skills, and attitudes throughout their careers. Many professional organizations mandate continuous education in regulation, licensure, and codes of ethics. As a result, safety and provision of optimal care and service for individuals, communities, and society as a whole depend on the critical appraisal and application of new information that will confirm, modify, and alter professional practice.

Definitions and History

Research literacy is an evolving subject, one that has emerged in response to our era of technological and knowledge explosions and an expanding emphasis on evidence-informed models of health and community practice (Jakubec, 2015). Box 1.1 explores the definitions and history of the concept of research literacy as it relates to health and community practice.

In an *evidence-informed practice model*, the practitioner bases treatment decisions on a blend of information gleaned from research evidence, patient values, and practitioner expertise and skills (Sackett, Strauss, Richardson, Rosenberg & Haynes, 2000). Patient and practitioner preferences as well as peer group advice are also found to influence decision making (Gabbay & le May, 2004). Fundamental to evidence-informed practice is not only the existence or creation of relevant research evidence, but also the ability of students and interprofessional practitioners to evaluate the literature and research papers in a critical and informed manner. A process of defining problems and questions; searching, appraising, and synthesizing the available research evidence; and adapting, implementing, and evaluating best evidence for practice is identified as "evidence-informed decision making" (National Collaborating Centre for Methods and Tools, 2016, "STEPS," para. 2). This process is illustrated in figure 1.1, a process referred to further in this textbook.

In this process, a truly evidence-informed practice approach depends on the creation of research-literate practitioners; *research-literate* is defined as understanding research language and its application to practice (Nolan & Behi,

Box 1.1: Definitions and History—Research Literacy

Research literacy is an essential competency for evidence-informed practice. It is the ability to locate, understand, and critically evaluate evidence for application in practice (Nolan & Behi, 1996). This topic is distinct from *research capacity*, which is the ability to *conduct* research (Fitchett, Tartaglia, Dodd-McCue & Murphy, 2012; Wayne et al., 2008; Williamson, 2007).

Research literacy is considered a component of "research mindedness," which includes the following features:

- Comprehension of the significance and relationship of research to practice
- Abilities to draw on research to inform practice
- Awareness of various research approaches and strategies
- Appreciation of the strengths and limitations of different research methods
- Critical and open-minded appraisal of research findings and literature (Maidment, Chilvers, Crichton-Hill & Meadows-Taurua, 2011)

The following skills are instrumental to research literacy:

1. Formulating researchable questions
2. Accessing information from multiple sources
3. Differentiating which information to consider as evidence
4. Critically evaluating and synthesizing evidence
5. Interpreting evidence to make clinical judgments
6. Incorporating research findings into communications with colleagues, patients, and community groups
7. Maintaining ethical, responsible, and compassionate standards of practice
8. Routine reflection on practice from multiple perspectives
9. Participation in the culture of research (Kreitzer, Sierpina & Fleishman, 2010)

In summary, the basic competencies of research literacy are the abilities to find, understand, critically appraise, and apply the evidence for practice.

Source: Adapted from "Research Literacy," by S.L. Jakubec, 2015, in M.J. Smith, R. Carpenter & J.J. Fitzpatrick (Eds.), *Encyclopedia of Nursing Education*, pp. 297–299, New York, NY: Springer. Adapted with permission.

1996; Williams, 2002). The task of becoming a research-literate practitioner is important in many ways, as it will enable you to do the following:

- Be conversant in the process of evidence-informed decision making, which supports your ability to communicate with other professionals and clients.
- Remain current, reflective, critical, and responsive in your work.
- Make the best possible choices and provide the best possible care or interventions to clients.
- Be a better consumer and an advocate of the best use of health care resources.

Figure 1.1: Evidence-Informed Decision-Making Process Model

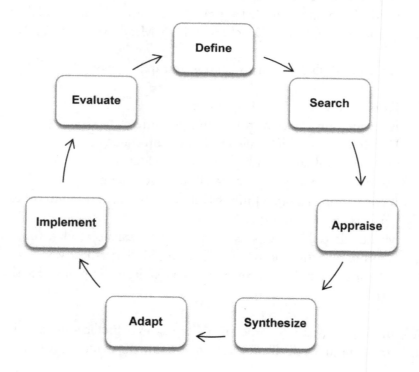

Source: Adapted from *Evidence-Informed Public Health,* by National Collaborating Centre for Methods and Tools, 2016, Hamilton, Canada: McMaster University. Copyright 2016 by McMaster University. Adapted with permission.

OBJECTIVES OF THE TEXT AND CHAPTER SUMMARIES

The aim of this textbook is to introduce students and interprofessional practitioners to the key concepts and activities involved in research literacy. Our intent in introducing research is twofold:

1. To enable you to better understand the research you read to inform your practice and to make some judgments about the quality of the research available.
2. To prepare you to undertake research utilization and knowledge translation (see chapters 8 and 9), either as part of your role at work or in more advanced academic study and research.

Many students and interprofessional practitioners believe that understanding research and using and mobilizing knowledge for practice are beyond their scope. Many are also intimidated by the new language and process of evidence-informed practice. This textbook addresses these fears and demystifies the complexities by demonstrating that the processes involved in the design and undertaking of research are easily understood. In this chapter (chapter 1), we introduced you to the background and definitions of research literacy in health and community practice, and the practical concerns for acquiring greater literacy. Next, chapter 2 focuses on understanding what knowledge and evidence are, and how *research* and *evidence* are distinguished from other forms of information or knowledge. Chapter 3 more specifically describes how a research study is different from other forms of knowledge and evidence. You will be introduced to the processes that a researcher might go through in order to generate a research question as a way of appreciating how research begins, and how your everyday practice could inspire research questions. Chapter 3 also introduces some of the philosophical assumptions that underpin research, including those that inform the quantitative and qualitative paradigms. In addition, ethical considerations in research are addressed, such as exploring the key ethical principles and ideas that inform all phases of the research process.

Chapter 4 focuses on how to search for information and research evidence in order to access and experience knowledge in a practical way. You will be guided in advanced techniques for database and keyword searching, referencing, organizing, and other information literacy skills. We will also provide an overview of the task of writing a literature review. In this era of information overload, understanding these techniques is critical to accessing current evidence that you can apply in your practice. Chapter 5 broadly explores how research papers are critically appraised. The general anatomy of a research paper is discussed, as are generic steps of writing a research critique.

Chapter 6 explores how to understand and interpret qualitative research papers. This includes assisting you to understand qualitative research goals, qualitative research questions, and the ways data are gathered, organized, interpreted, and analyzed. Chapter 6 also provides an introduction to some primary qualitative research methodologies and methods, the questions they are intent on answering, as well as the sampling methods and the key methods (data collection tools). You will move from the general understanding of critical appraisal to being able to interpret the findings in a qualitative study (e.g., the thematic or narrative analyses presented), appraise the research, and learn how to reference qualitative research for practice.

Chapter 7 explores how to understand and interpret quantitative research papers. This includes assisting you to understand quantitative research goals, quantitative research questions, and the ways in which data are gathered, organized, interpreted, and analyzed. You will be introduced to some of the primary quantitative research methodologies and some research methods. You will move from a general understanding of critical appraisals to being able to interpret the results (e.g., basic descriptive or correlations statistics) in a quantitative research paper, appraise the research, and learn how to reference quantitative research for practice. This chapter also discusses the need to employ mixed methodologies and methods in research for health and community practice in order to gain a more holistic view of some of the complex issues found in practice.

Chapter 8 responds to the questions: How do I know what is best evidence? How do I know if research in practice (i.e., policies and guidelines) is current and the best available evidence? In this chapter, you will have an opportunity to reflect on how best evidence can be adapted for practice, policies, and guidelines.

Chapter 9 addresses how to use research in practice. In this chapter, you will integrate the skills you have learned from the preceding chapters in order to address how research can be implemented and evaluated in your practice. Specifically, you will explore how the concepts of knowledge translation and knowledge utilization are mobilized and applied to practice.

The final section of this textbook includes a collection of supplemental materials: further resources and links, an expanded glossary, practice exam questions, and practical learning activities that you may find useful.

DESCRIPTION OF WAYS TO APPROACH AND USE THE TEXT

With the ongoing need to have the best research-based evidence to address various issues in health and community disciplines, it is imperative that students and interprofessional practitioners possess a foundational understanding of how to access, read, and appraise research, and then take this information and apply it in their own processes and approaches at a level appropriate for their scope of practice (Melnyk

& Fineout-Overholt, 2015). The overall goal of *Research Literacy for Health and Community Practice* is to support students and practitioners to understand research *for* practice, which entails learning basic research literacy knowledge and skills to search, interpret and understand, and appraise and use research effectively in practice.

At various points within each chapter you can break to complete one of the practical learning activities and review other resources (see appendix B). Undertaking the practical learning activities is an important element of your understanding of the content of each chapter. As well, select chapters will have a Research in Practice box example. Engaging in activity-based learning opportunities appears to be effective in improving research knowledge and critical appraisal abilities (see box 1.2).

Box 1.2: Research in Practice—A Review of the Evidence on Improving Research Literacy

This systematic review of the literature sought to identify the most effective workplace and educational interventions designed for improving nurses' understanding and critical use of the research literature. Through a broad search of relevant research, 10 of 96 papers met the criteria and found that activity-based learning and programs with a strong base in theory were most effective in supporting research literacy. The study recommends these approaches when planning educational programs in order to improve research knowledge, critical appraisal, and research self-efficacy. The inquiry also recommends more rigorous study of educational interventions on research literacy and evidence-informed practice.

Source: "The Effectiveness of Interventions for Improving the Research Literacy of Nurses: A Systematic Review," by S. Hines, J. Ramsbotham & F. Coyer, 2015, *Worldviews on Evidence-Based Nursing, 12,* pp. 265–272. Copyright 2015 by Hines et al. Reprinted with permission.

You are encouraged, where appropriate, to reflect on other theories and courses you may have taken or are taking, and how the things you have learned from working in health or community practice also inform your understanding of research. Other activities will require you to take time away from the textbook to refer to or find out new information that will add to your understanding of the topic under discussion. Some activities challenge you to apply your learning to a question or scenario to help you think about a theme in more depth in order to add to your understanding. A few activities require you to make observations during your day-to-day life or practice. All these activities are designed to increase your understanding of the topics under discussion and how they reflect on practice. We recommend that, where possible, you try to engage with the practical learning activities, or as instructed by your professors or team leaders, in order to increase your understanding of the realities of research for practice.

Other features of the textbook you will work with include the Learning Objectives section highlighted at the start of each chapter and the Review and Reflect summaries at the conclusion of each chapter. Additional resources of interest and exam review questions are provided for each chapter (see appendix A). The keywords that appear in each chapter are described both in the text and in the glossary. As in any language course, learning this new lexicon becomes central to your literacy (in this case research literacy) and to using research in practice.

REVIEW AND REFLECT

There are three main points in understanding research literacy:

1. Research literacy is distinct from research capacity or abilities to conduct research. Rather, research literacy is concerned with the understanding and application of research for practice.
2. Research literacy is considered a part of *research mindedness*, an essential competency for evidence-informed health and community practice. Skills of research literacy include formulating researchable questions, accessing information, differentiating which information to consider as evidence, critically evaluating and synthesizing evidence, interpreting evidence to make clinical judgments, referencing research in communications with others, maintaining ethical standards in all practices, expressing habits of reflection drawing on multiple perspectives to enhance clinical practice, and participating in the culture of research.
3. Research literacy has been studied across a number of disciplines and among students at all levels—it is an essential competency for all health and community practice fields. In this textbook, research literacy is approached much like learning a language. The basic building blocks of the language are explored here, with a view toward expanding your knowledge and skills for an everyday fluency in the language of research. Use of the text features and accompanying practical learning activities will strengthen your understanding of research literacy.

2 | WHAT ARE KNOWLEDGE AND EVIDENCE?

"We are drowning in information but starved for knowledge."

—John Naisbitt

LEARNING OBJECTIVES

This chapter focuses on understanding what knowledge and evidence are and how research and evidence are distinguished from other forms of information or knowledge. After reading this chapter and completing the practical learning activities in appendix B, you will be able to do the following:

- Describe how we know what we know.
- Describe distinct forms of knowledge.
- Distinguish between information and information literacy.
- Explain what is considered to be evidence and how evidence is formulated through research.
- Describe researchable questions and the research process.

CHAPTER OUTLINE

- Knowledge
  - How Do We Know What We Know?
  - What Are Forms of Knowledge?
  - Practical and Professional Knowledge—Knowledge for Practice
- Information
  - What Is Information and Information Literacy?
- Evidence
  - What Is Evidence? Why Is It Important?
  - How Is Evidence Formulated through Research?
- Research
  - What Questions Do I See in Practice or Daily Life? What Constitutes a Research Question?
  - What Are Different Approaches to Different Questions? How Is an Inquiry Started?
  - What Are Researchable Questions and How Does a Question Shape the Kind of Evidence, Knowledge, and Information?
  - What Types of Research Questions Will Respond to Your Issues in Practice?
- Review and Reflect

KNOWLEDGE

We use the word "know" all the time—for instance, "I know that being late all the time creates a lot of social and work problems"—but what does it really mean to "know" something? Fortunately, the study of *knowledge* is something philosophers have wrestled with for centuries. The discipline is known as *epistemology*, which comes from the Greek words *episteme*, meaning "knowledge," and *logos*, meaning "reason." Epistemology literally means to reason about knowledge—the kinds of things we can know, the limits to what we can know, and even if it is possible to actually know anything at all! In order to answer that question, you probably have to have some idea what the term *know* means.

How Do We Know What We Know?

Often people claim to know and accept things as facts without question. There are lots of reasons for this sort of acceptance, but the most likely is that we have picked up a definition of *knowledge* over time and have a general sense of what the term means. Many of us would probably say that knowledge is something that is true and includes some of the following elements:

Certainty—it is hard if not impossible to deny.
Evidence—it is based on actual, traceable things.
Practicality—it has to actually work in the real world.
Broad agreement—many others agree it is true.

If you think about it, each of these elements of knowledge has problems. For example, what would you claim to know that you would also say you are certain of? What does "broad agreement" really involve? For instance, what would constitute agreement, and what would be broad enough agreement? In reality, there are many things we might claim to know that are not, or cannot be, broadly agreed upon. For example, suppose you are experiencing back pain. You might tell your health care practitioner that you know you are in pain. Unfortunately, only *you* can claim to know that (and, as an added problem, you don't appear to have any *evidence* for it either—you just feel a strong and intense sensation of pain). Based upon a verbal admission, it seems you may know things that do not have evidence to substantiate them, or have the broad agreement of others. These problems of what constitutes knowing something are among the interests of philosophers. These are the problems that make defining *knowledge* very challenging, making it difficult to answer the question, "How do we know what we know?"

What Are Forms of Knowledge?

The terms *explicit* and *tacit*, as well as *propositional* and *non-propositional*, are often used in relation to forms of knowledge. These terms are often summarized as *knowing that* and *knowing how*. The distinction between tacit and explicit knowledge is a fundamental concept to understand regarding research for practice and how to read research papers in your field of study or practice. Michael Polanyi first made the distinction between these forms of knowledge in the 1960s (Polanyi, 1968, 1998). *Explicit* or *propositional knowledge* is formal and systematic; it is knowledge that can be expressed in words and numbers, and can be easily communicated and shared. Conversely, *tacit* or *non-propositional knowledge* is described as something not easily visible and expressible. Tacit knowledge is highly personal, hard to formalize, and difficult to communicate. For example, subjective insights, intuitions, and hunches fall into this category of knowledge. It is deeply rooted in action and is captured in the term *know-how*. Tacit knowledge consists of mental models, beliefs, and perspectives so ingrained in our thinking that we take them for granted and, therefore, this form of knowledge is not easily shared in a structured way. In discussing this subject, Polanyi (1968) provided the example of riding a bicycle. The explicit knowledge for riding a bicycle might be a set of instructions such as this:

1. Stand beside your bike, hold both the handlebars, and look forward.
2. Walk briskly forward or run a few paces taking the bike with you.
3. Now mount the bike, putting one foot on each pedal.
4. Start pedalling while maintaining your balance and continue in this manner.

Do these instructions accurately express the knowledge or the skill of riding a bicycle? The actual knowledge comes through that "ah-ha" moment and the ability to repeat this knowledge without thinking. As a result, the more you practise riding a bike, the more confidence you gain. Such knowledge—for example, in step four above—is indeed difficult to put into words because it becomes embedded and used subconsciously.

In our current contexts of health and community practice, explicit or propositional knowledge is often considered to have a higher status than tacit or non-propositional knowledge. Non-propositional knowledge, *knowing how,* is experience-based knowledge, and includes professional craft knowledge and personal knowledge. This is particularly relevant in professional practice disciplines such as in the fields of health and social work.

Professional craft knowledge that is embedded in practice can be tacit (i.e., implied, understood, inferred) and includes both general professional knowledge gained from experience and specific knowledge related to a particular client, community, or situation. See box 2.1 for a summary of a study exploring tacit and explicit knowledge in the field of public health.

Professional knowledge is acquired from a variety of experiences (e.g., listening to clients, learning and implementing practice skills, reflection and clinical reasoning, and peer affiliation and mentorship). Propositional knowledge provides you with theory for which the values and experiences of your clients, communities, and colleagues can be reflected upon in decisions and practice. Non-propositional professional tacit knowledge enables you to use that theory in practice while providing additional (although unproven) evidence from practice. Personal knowledge allows a deeper understanding of the needs and issues within the context of practice, inviting more holistic approaches (Jones & Rivett, 2004).

Box 2.1: Research in Practice—Professional Knowledge in Public Health Practice: Tacit and Explicit

The premise of this exploratory research study is that public health practice is both a science and an art. In this qualitative narrative inquiry research study, one-on-one interviews and focus groups were conducted with practitioners from four public health units in order to gain a better understanding of how tacit knowledge is used to inform program initiatives in public health. The research found that tacit knowledge (specifically in practices of exploring opportunity, bringing teams together, and working out program details for partnering and funding) was used to plan public health initiatives. Tacit knowledge was found to draw from, and be embedded within, various stages of program planning of public health.

Source: "The Use of Tacit and Explicit Knowledge in Public Health: A Qualitative Study," by A. Kothari et al., 2012, *Implementation Science, 7*(20). Copyright 2012 by Kothari et al.

Practical and Professional Knowledge—Knowledge for Practice

Personal knowledge is shaped by our individual life experiences and is, therefore, unique to every health and community practitioner. This includes the collective knowledge of the individual practitioner's community and culture and one's personal values, assumptions, beliefs, and attitudes. Personal knowledge creates the basis for our interpersonal interactions. Personal knowledge helps us to determine what has meaning for clients and communities, which is an essential element in practice. In order to be effective and responsive practitioners, we need multiple types of knowledge from a wide variety of sources.

The knowledge base found in professional practice is one of the defining characteristics of professions and is essential for sound reasoning and decision making (Higgs, Jones & Titchen, 2008). All health and community practitioners, including nurses, midwives, physicians, social workers, occupational therapists, or other professionals, spend a considerable amount of time gaining the necessary knowledge to practise their chosen careers. All of these professions encourage a strong commitment to lifelong learning. This approach is required to build upon the entry-level knowledge base, which is necessary to move from a novice to an experienced practitioner (Jensen, Gwyer, Hack & Shepard, 2007).

Knowledge is dynamic, and knowledge in any one category can be translated into another category. All of these types of knowledge are modified through practice—combined, extended, collapsed, and made specific to address the realities of the context (Higgs, Fish & Rothwell, 2008). It is the process of practical reasoning that facilitates the integration of all these types of knowledge (Edwards & Jones, 2007). Activity 2.1 in appendix B guides you through a reflection on the different types of knowledge on a topic of your interest.

INFORMATION

Facts, data, figures, details, advice, wisdom, and stories are just some of the information entering your everyday world through images, text, audio, video, and other sources. In our era of information overload, we must be able to sift through information in an efficient and thoughtful way; there is simply too much information available to be useful and make sense of it otherwise! It is important to note that information, unto itself, cannot be considered knowledge or evidence, and, as will be discussed further in chapter 3, data and facts are meaningless unless they are situated in a theoretical context. Information must be filtered through our experiences, then applied and reflected upon to become meaningful, otherwise it remains just data. Information and data must be gathered, read, assembled, observed, questioned, conceptualized, judged, manipulated, integrated, analyzed, synthesized, and evaluated before they become knowledge (Hayden, 2013) and, as discussed later in this chapter, a formal and systematic process must be followed before it is considered research.

What Is Information and Information Literacy?

There are numerous definitions of information literacy available (CILIP Information Literacy Group, 2014). Briefly, *information literacy* is considered the set of learning and critical thinking skills necessary to access, evaluate, and use information effectively and efficiently (Julien & Boon, 2004). Whether for completing an assignment or working in health and community practice, information literacy means discerning the most appropriate way to search for needed information, and understanding that *information* is different from *knowledge*.

EVIDENCE

What Is Evidence? Why Is It Important?

The origins of the term *evidence* reside in legal discourse, in which lawyers might talk about material proof in a court case. In health and community practice, evidence is also understood as it relates to proof of rationality, or information that has stood up to scrutiny by way of methods, such as observation or other systematic techniques (Rycroft-Malone et al., 2004).

What is important in the use of language for this textbook is understanding *what counts* as evidence in terms of evidence-informed practice. As indicated in table 2.1, there are three essential differences between research and evidence-informed practice. Although both are systematic, each has a different purpose. Research is used to conduct an investigation in order to generate results that will add to existing evidence. On the other hand, evidence-informed practice aims to search for and appraise the best evidence, some of which will be found in research (as discussed in chapter 1), as well as the inclusion of a practitioner's judgment and client values. Rycroft-Malone et al. (2004) and others (e.g., Greenhalgh, 2014; National Research Council, 2012) reflect on the ways research, with certain hierarchies, is the best form of evidence for decision making, to the exclusion of a more complete view of thoughtful decision making for practice. These critiques and the distinction between research *producing* evidence and evidence-informed practice are further emphasized here.

An important distinction between research and evidence-informed practice is seen in their outcomes. In research, the outcome is specified at the beginning of the study, such as the goal of exploring the relationships between variables, providing a description or exploration of current practice, or of testing a particular hypothesis or theory. The goals of research may or may not result in recommendations for changes in practice. However, the outcome of evidence-informed practice is to make clinical decisions, which may include changing practice. Differences between research and evidence-informed practice are listed in table 2.1.

How Is Evidence Formulated through Research?

The term *research* is often used in advertising, sometimes correctly and sometimes incorrectly. How often do you hear the expression, "Research tells us ..."? Before going any further, pause to think about what is meant by research. For the purposes of this textbook, *research* is one form of evidence for practice decision making: it is a systematic, planned investigation of a specified problem that will contribute to understanding the phenomena in question. Thus, a research project begins with identifying a problem to be investigated and ends with an outcome in the form of results and recommendations (Carnwell, 2001).

Although research involves information gathering, simply collecting information from multiple sources and putting it together is not research. Ask, what information would make you confident in responding to a problem in practice.

Table 2.1: Differences between Research and Evidence-Informed Practice

	Research	Evidence-Informed Practice
Process	Systematic and planned	Systematic search and investigation appraisal of best evidence
Purpose	Specification of a problem to be investigated	Use of evidence for making clinical decisions to be investigated
Goal/Objective	Statement of predetermined outcome (e.g., results of the patient as well as research recommendations)	Account taken of individual needs of the patient as well as evidence-informed evidence
Outcome	Contribute to understanding	Bring about changes in practice

What would help you choose a solution and think you can use this in your practice? To answer this question, data must be systematically gathered, critically examined, and analyzed in order to be considered research evidence.

Researchers should follow this process:

- Identify an issue or problem and develop a topic that is turned into a research question.
- Situate the work within the existing literature by conducting a literature review (see chapter 4).
- State a clear purpose of the research.
- Decide the aims, objectives, approach, or theoretical perspective to guide their research as well as the design (including methods such as observations, surveys, or interviews).
- Obtain ethical approval for the study if involving human subjects (see chapter 3).
- Collect, analyze, and interpret the data.
- Evaluate and report on the research findings.

RESEARCH

What Questions Do I See in Practice or Daily Life? What Constitutes a Research Question?

To begin, there are always research questions waiting to be answered in your practice and everyday life. Consider what sorts of things fascinate you. For example, you may be curious about the ways globalization impacts mental health. Activity 2.2 in appendix B guides you through issues, problem, sub-problem, and research question explorations.

No topic or issue is without controversy. We all have different views and opinions, but it is the task of researchers to evaluate the existing knowledge base and apply the rules of scientific research to identify gaps. Once information of the existing knowledge base has been collected, researchers can begin to better understand a question within the context of others' work. This process of searching and reviewing the literature is discussed in more detail in chapter 4. Typically, researchers follow a literature review by setting forth their research question. Research questions move the knowledge forward—they do not just replicate what someone else has done before, but instead offer something new. Depending on the goals of a research study, researchers may state the research question as a hypothesis by posing a prediction of what they think they will find, and then will test that hypothesis to see if it holds true (e.g., children who have less screen time will have higher test scores). Often researchers will simply state the general question they seek to answer without offering a hypothesis (e.g., is screen time associated with lower test scores?). The research question should be both clearly stated and answered by the end of the research paper.

What Are Different Approaches to Different Questions? How Is an Inquiry Started?

The starting point for all research is uncertainty (Ellis, 2013). In the case of research, uncertainty is not a bad thing. A lack of certainty in an area is what initiates a question to study. Uncertainty emerges in all areas of health and social disciplines, from questioning whether a treatment will be effective for a particular condition to understanding what it is like to recover from substance use disorders while living on the streets. Research questions may develop in response to social, environmental, or political situations, or may arise from new ideas that emerge from research or practice. To follow are some examples of ways that health and community practitioners become aware of issues they want to explore:

- At a community health conference, a women's group suggested increased rates of sexual assault in communities where health, social support, policing, and legal or prosecution services did not have a formalized team approach.
- Data from a national health survey revealed increasing rates of workplace injuries.
- A community group noted a lack of access to recreation and social linkages for seniors in suburban neighbourhoods, particularly for those who were new immigrants or did not speak English.
- The provincial government announced a promise to improve mental health care in remote and isolated communities.

Given that the starting point for research is uncertainty, where do we move to next? Briefly, there is a need to frame research questions that are relevant to the problem or issue being considered and that are also able to address the uncertainty raised.

Why is research important then? If we cannot guarantee that research can answer the questions we pose, why do it? Any research is only as good as the methodologies and methods it employs. All research papers present a specific methodology and systematic, structured design of study. A research methodology and implementation of that design is what distinguishes a research paper from editorials, discussion papers, or other such contributions to knowledge. Chapters 6 and 7 of this textbook will introduce you to the more common methodologies and guide you on how to appraise specific qualitative, quantitative, and mixed-methods research papers. The aim is to equip you with the tools not only to read and understand research in these areas, but also to think about how and why research is important to your health and community practice.

What Are Researchable Questions and How Does a Question Shape the Kind of Evidence, Knowledge, and Information?

The type of question is important and can help lead you to the best research papers to appraise and review to understand your issues and problems in practice. According to Springett and Campbell (2006), developing the right question is absolutely crucial to the rest of the research process: "Getting the right answer to the wrong question is going to waste an awful lot of time and resources. However, the main problem is not asking the wrong question, but not properly defining the right question" (p. 26).

By carefully considering the questions you have for your issues in practice, you can think like a researcher and focus in on the kinds of research studies that might inform your practice. It may take time upfront, but will save time and effort later on in your work—whether that work is for an assignment or in your practice. For example, if you are working in a field with people experiencing eating disorders, you may ask yourself a number of important questions about the topic, such as, "What causes eating disorders?" In this case, you will need to define the topic further—ask yourself what specific eating disorder and what sort of terms, definitions, and classifications you are curious about (e.g., anorexia nervosa, bulimia, binge eating disorder, and so on). You will also need to further define the terms of your own questions, which can help you decipher the terms you will need to search and understand from the existing literature. For example, you may want to decide if the "cause" is in fact what you are curious about, or if you can even discover a cause. Or perhaps what "influences" eating disorders is more relevant to your practice issues. Therefore, if the research question you are interested in is, "What factors influence eating disorders?," you still may need to narrow to a specific population or point in time in treatment or other delimiting terms. You may then revise the question you will explore as, "What factors influence the beginning or development of eating disorders?" Of course, within this one topic, there are many questions that might and have been studied. You could indeed seek to uncover other questions about eating disorders:

- Why do eating disorders occur?
- How many kinds of eating disorders are there?
- Who develops eating disorders?
- Where do eating disorders occur most often (geographical distribution or patterns)?
- What treatments are available for people with eating disorders?
- When do eating disorders start?

What Types of Research Questions Will Respond to Your Issues in Practice?
Any number of research questions will guide your literature search, and assist you in responding to issues or questions in your practice. You begin by focusing on your topic, defining the terms of what you want to understand, and operationalizing or defining the boundaries of what you want to better understand. Clearly defining the research question or problem (see figure 2.1) is an important point of entry into the process of evidence-informed decision making introduced in chapter 1.

You can then focus on questions to which you seek answers in your search of the existing literature, narrow those questions, and experiment further. This will enable you to broadly inform your topic or problem, and perhaps specifically respond to your question (e.g., the question of what the best choice of therapy may be for an individual from a particular age group). Table 2.2 shows some of the common types of questions you may find in practice and the types of studies that begin to examine the questions. In activity 2.1 in appendix B, you will have an opportunity to explore some of the ways to consider questions in your field of interest. Additional types of studies will be further elaborated in subsequent chapters.

Figure 2.1: The Define Step in the Evidence-Informed Decision-Making Process

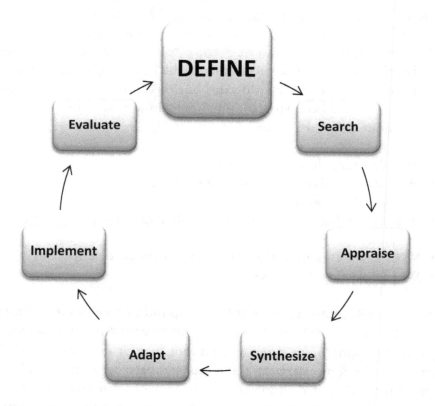

Source: Adapted from *Evidence-Informed Public Health*, by National Collaborating Centre for Methods and Tools, 2016, Hamilton, Canada: McMaster University. Copyright 2016 by McMaster University. Adapted with permission.

Table 2.2: Common Types of Research Questions

Common Questions in Health and Community Practice	Type of Research Study
How can we select the best intervention that will do more good than harm or that will be cost-effective?	Intervention study
How can we understand what is going on (such as how many people hold certain views, live in certain conditions, etc.)?	Descriptive study
How can we determine if two or more variables (e.g., gender and treatment outcome, spiritual beliefs and perspectives on a social issue, etc.) relate to one another?	Relational study
How can we identify the causes for a disease or social problem?	Causal (harm or risk) study
How can we estimate the likelihood over time of anticipated disease or complications?	Prognosis study

REVIEW AND REFLECT

There is no end to the issues and problems you may want to explore for health and community practice. As you review research evidence to inform your practice, look for a clearly identified research question and a formal research process. Questions asked by the researcher will shape the development of a research study and influence the research process. The research process includes a clear research problem or purpose, literature review, an identified theoretical perspective and design (including methods such as observations, surveys, or interviews), and ethical approval sought. The formal research process will include a report on data collected, analyzed, and interpreted along with a discussion of the research findings and results.

3 | HOW IS RESEARCH FRAMED AND ORGANIZED, AND HOW ARE ETHICS APPLIED?

"I like the scientific spirit—the holding off, the being sure but not too sure, the willingness to surrender ideas when the evidence is against them: this is ultimately fine—it always keeps the way beyond open—always gives life, thought, affection, the whole man, a chance to try over again after a mistake—after a wrong guess."

—Walt Whitman

LEARNING OBJECTIVES

All research is based on some underlying assumptions and theories about what constitutes "valid" research, and which research methods are appropriate for the development of knowledge in a study. Your research literacy depends on your knowledge of what these assumptions are. This chapter discusses the philosophical assumptions that relate to knowledge making and reasoning (deductive and inductive) and explains the design strategies of qualitative and quantitative approaches to research. It explores how knowledge is framed and organized, as well as the paradigms and frameworks for knowledge formation. After reading this chapter and completing the practical learning activities in appendix B, you will be able to do the following:

- Describe how different assumptions, beliefs, and theories guide the research studies that can inform your practice.
- Understand the difference between deductive and inductive reasoning and between quantitative, qualitative, and mixed-methods research paradigms.
- Explain how ethical principles are applied in research.

CHAPTER OUTLINE

- What Are Paradigms, Theory, Research, and Data?
- How Do Paradigms Shape Research Questions and Research?
  - Deductive and Inductive Reasoning
- Classifying Research Paradigms
  - The Quantitative Research Paradigm
  - The Qualitative Research Paradigm
  - The Mixed-Methods Research Paradigm
- How Are Ethics Applied in Research?
  - Research with Human Subjects
  - Research with Animal Subjects
- Review and Reflect

WHAT ARE PARADIGMS, THEORY, RESEARCH, AND DATA?

A *paradigm* may be seen as a set of assumptions and beliefs that cannot be determined to be true or false; rather it represents a pattern, view, or example of something. Were we able to prove or disprove paradigms, as Guba and Lincoln (1994) state, "The philosophical debates ... would have been resolved millennia ago" (pp. 107–108). Holding a particular worldview, however, influences personal behaviours, professional practice, and the perspectives taken by others in a relationship. Ultimately, holding one worldview or another will influence the positions taken as to how theories or ideas of how things work relate to one another. Research paradigms in this way "define for the [researcher] what it is they are about, and what falls within and outside the limits of [research]" (Guba & Lincoln, 1994, p. 108). Testing theories and exploring the evidence that may support a broader view of what is occurring is the overarching task of the research process. Clarity of the elements for knowledge making in the research process is called *data* (Bouma, Ling & Wilkinson, 2012).

While data are thought to be empirical facts, in and of themselves facts and data are meaningless. The facts (e.g., data gathered about lung capacity and body weight before, during, and after a treadmill desk intervention) only obtain meaning when related to theories (e.g., in the treadmill intervention, these might be theories about how sedentary work influences physical health). Data are the actual words or measurements taken in a study to test the hypothesis. As Bouma et al. (2012) noted, these kinds of data can be classified as quantitative or qualitative, which respond to different kinds of questions relating to understanding issues of quantity (e.g., How much? How many? How often?) and quality (e.g., What is it like? What is going on? What is the experience?).

HOW DO PARADIGMS SHAPE RESEARCH QUESTIONS AND RESEARCH?

To explore the issues with which you are concerned, you need to organize your thoughts and ideas. It is important to apply reasoning processes and appropriate kinds of questions in order to arrive at reasonable conclusions in a study that may inform your practice. It is the same whether you are a researcher or a curious inquirer in your health and community practice. Regardless of your research activity (producing or consuming), bring curiosity, skepticism, and reasoning to how you work with research. We often refer to the two broad methods of reasoning as the *deductive* and *inductive* approaches.

Deductive and Inductive Reasoning

If you use *deductive* reasoning, you explore a general idea and then try to draw particular conclusions. Informally, this is called a "top-down" approach (Trochim, 2006). This approach begins by proposing a theory regarding your topic of interest for your study. You then narrow that issue down into more specific hypotheses that can be tested, and then collect observations to address the hypotheses. Testing the hypotheses with specific data as a confirmation (or not) of the original theories results in a particular kind of deductive knowledge development (see figure 3.1). Certain issues and problems lend themselves to this sort of knowledge development and reasoning. For instance, based on the process presented in figure 3.1, consider how you would use deductive reasoning to explore the issue of obesity or the issue of urban street gang affiliation.

Figure 3.1: The Deductive Approach to Research

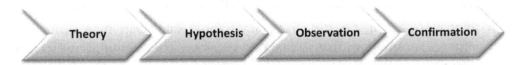

Inductive reasoning works the other way, moving from specific observations to broader generalizations and theories. Informally, we sometimes call this a "bottom-up" approach (Trochim, 2006). In inductive reasoning, we start with specific observations and measures, begin to detect patterns and regularities, formulate some tentative hypotheses that can be explored, and finally develop some general conclusions or theories. Consider how you would use inductive reasoning to explore the issues of obesity or urban street gang affiliation, and how you might approach research on these phenomena based on the inductive approach to research represented in figure 3.2.

Figure 3.2: The Inductive Approach to Research

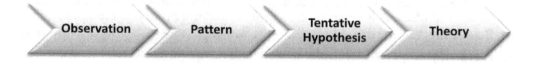

These two methods of reasoning lead to distinctly different approaches to research questions. Inductive reasoning, by its very nature, is more open-ended and exploratory, especially at the beginning. Deductive reasoning is narrower in scope and is concerned with testing or confirming hypotheses. Even though a particular study may look purely deductive (e.g., an experiment designed to test the hypothesized effects of a treatment on some outcome), most research in health and community practice involves both inductive and deductive reasoning processes at some time in the project. Even in the most constrained experiment, the researchers may observe patterns in the data that lead them to develop new theories (Shtarkshall, 2004). In this way, these two research approaches rely on one another to generate knowledge that makes sense in practice (we discuss this further in chapters 6 and 7). Indeed, both deductive and inductive reasoning are critical to the research process. The ultimate goal is to logically connect ideas and explain discoveries through theory (so we simply do not just have facts). Theories help us to explain the relationship between variables.

CLASSIFYING RESEARCH PARADIGMS

The emphasis of the questions asked in practice and research helps us in identifying the nature or assumptions that will guide a response. These assumptions lead to very distinct forms of research outcomes. In research terminology, this means you need to identify the paradigm within which your question sits.

Simply put, paradigms are the philosophical basis of the question being asked, the nature of the study needed to address the question that has been identified. In health and community practice research, as in most practical research, we commonly identify three major research paradigms: quantitative, qualitative, and mixed methods (Creswell, 2014). These paradigms refer to distinctly different ways of viewing the world and provide different responses and approaches to research questions, offering different research outcomes (see table 3.1).

The Quantitative Research Paradigm

The quantitative paradigm is the one you might most associate with scientific ways of thinking. It involves viewing the world in ways that are measurable or provable. The quantitative element of the paradigm refers to the ability of research within this paradigm to quantify findings. In other words, the findings can be counted or can be demonstrated in a way that is measurable.

Quantitative research is concerned with proof, cause and effect, and demonstrating associations between variables (Locke, Silverman & Spirduso, 2010). Quantitative research often starts with a hypothesis, an idea yet to be tested using established scientific methods. Chapter 7 explores the approaches to research that fall within this research paradigm. Data collection within the quantitative paradigm is deductive. That is, quantitative research starts with a hypothesis or idea that it seeks to confirm or refute. Deductive reasoning follows predetermined methods for collecting data. Deductive research works from general observations toward a more specific outcome, and in this respect it is considered to be "knowledge driven." Deductive research is about things we think we know, such as subjects and objects we can see and quantify. Its primary purpose is to prove or disprove areas of perceived knowledge. Consider, then, how quantitative perspectives may frame research questions about the earlier issues you reflected upon: obesity or the urban street gang affiliation. What sort of quantitative questions might be asked on these topics? Activity 3.1 in appendix B provides you with further opportunities to consider the ways different research paradigms would frame and respond to different questions from your interest or field of practice.

The Qualitative Research Paradigm

The qualitative paradigm is the one that you might most associate with the social sciences and people-centred methods of enquiry. It is a way of looking at the world from the point of view of people. It enquires about what people feel, think, understand, and believe. The qualitative paradigm is not so concerned with proof; rather, this method seeks to describe and understand human experiences from the point of view of the people who have had, or are currently having, the experience (Locke et al., 2010). Qualitative research is by its very nature inductive. That is, it generates ideas and theories from what is observed during the research.

The *qualitative* element of the paradigm refers to the fact that it seeks to understand things that cannot readily be measured or counted. It is more concerned with the quality of an experience, of meaning, understanding, and belief. Consider again the issues of obesity and urban street gangs—what sort of qualitative questions might be asked of these topics? Qualitative research starts with a question, something that needs to be explored; it may be used to generate a hypothesis, but it does not necessarily start with one. The data collected leads to the generation of ideas or hypotheses (hypotheses tested in deductive studies, as discussed above, are sometimes derived from inductive research). Researchers begin a study not knowing what they will find; they allow the data collected to lead them to the creation of a new idea or hypothesis. Chapter 6 explores the methodologies and approaches to research used within this paradigm.

The Mixed-Methods Research Paradigm

Mixed-methods research involves paradigm characteristics of both quantitative and qualitative methods (Tashakkori & Teddlie, 2010). In chapter 7, you will review the two major types of mixed research: mixed-method and mixed-model research. For now, keep in mind that the mixing of quantitative and qualitative research can take many forms. In fact, the possibilities for mixing are almost infinite.

The researcher should blend quantitative and qualitative research methods, procedures, and paradigm characteristics in such a way that the resulting mixture or combination has complementary strengths, without compounding any weaknesses (Tashakkori & Teddlie, 2010). The use of multiple methods or approaches to research ideally works in this way. When different approaches are used to focus on the same phenomenon and they provide the same result, you have corroboration of evidence that will strengthen the results (Creswell, 2014). Other important reasons for doing mixed research are to complement one set of results with another, to expand a set of results, or to discover something that would have been missed if only a quantitative or only a qualitative approach had been used.

The three paradigms offer different approaches to knowledge making and to responding to questions in your practice. Table 3.1 summarizes the differences in their respective *methodologies,* the general framework of the studies. These differences will be explored in further detail in chapters 6 and 7.

An important element of research literacy includes understanding what theories might be used to explore the questions in a research study. As illustrated in table 3.1, when employing quantitative methods, researchers often test theories as an explanation for answers to their questions. In qualitative methods, the use of theory is more varied and a researcher may generate a theory as the final outcome of a study.

Table 3.1: Distinct Assumptions and Approaches of Quantitative, Qualitative, and Mixed-Methods Research Paradigms

Element of Research Approach	Quantitative Paradigm	Qualitative Paradigm	Mixed-Methods Paradigm
Scientific method	Deductive (or top-down) approach	Inductive (or bottom-up) approach	Both deductive and inductive
Common research objectives	Description, explanation, prediction	Description, exploration, discovery	Multiple objectives
Focus	Narrow view, testing specific hypotheses	A wide and deep view; examining the breadth and depth of a phenomena, experience, or organization	Multiple foci
Perspective on human behaviour	Behaviour is regular and predictable	Behaviour is fluid, dynamic, situational, social, contextual, and personal	Behaviour is somewhat predictable
Nature of reality	Objective (different observers agree upon what is being seen)	Subjective, personal, and socially constructed	Common sense, realistic, and pragmatic, "what works"
Nature of observation	Attempt to study under controlled conditions	Study occurs in natural environments with attention to contextual realities	Study in more than one context or condition

(continued)

Table 3.1 (continued)

Nature of data	Variables	Words, images, and categories	Mixture of variables, words, and images
Form of data collected	Collect quantitative data based on precise measurements using structured and validated measures and instruments (e.g., closed-ended items, rating scales, codified behavioural responses)	Collect qualitative data (in-depth interviews, participant observation, field notes, open-ended questions); the researcher is the primary data-collection instrument	Multiple forms
Data analysis	Identify statistical relationships	Search for patterns, themes, and holistic features	Quantitative and qualitative
Results	Generalizable findings	Particularistic findings, representation of insider viewpoint, present multiple perspectives	Corroborated findings may generalize
Form of final report	Statistical report	Narrative report with contextual description with direct quotations from research participants	Eclectic and pragmatic reporting

In the qualitative research methodology called *grounded theory*, the place of theory is more central to the lens that shapes what is being studied and the questions asked. When utilizing mixed-methods approaches, researchers may both test theories and generate them. Mixed-methods research may contain a theoretical lens, such as a focus on feminist, racial, or class issues, that guides the entire study (Creswell, 2014).

You also may, as a practitioner, have a particular preference for one type of approach to research questions over another. If you do, how would this preference affect your connection to research in your health and community practice setting? If your topic or question in practice commands one type of approach, you will direct your search toward research in the corresponding paradigm. However, multiple understandings of an issue can also strengthen the holistic picture of what can be understood.

HOW ARE ETHICS APPLIED IN RESEARCH?

Ethics refers to a system of moral values or the way people distinguish right from wrong. Various international and national ethics governing bodies require all members to adhere to international codes of ethics, which apply to the treatment of both humans and animals (World Health Organization, 2016).

In the past, researchers performed all kinds of questionable experiments in the name of science. For example, in one famous experiment, psychologist Stanley Milgram led his subjects to believe that they would potentially be giving painful electric shocks to other people (Milgram, 1963). Many people considered this experiment unethical because it caused the subjects significant emotional discomfort. As another example, the medical research undertaken in Germany in the 1940s by the Nazis on unsuspecting prisoners of war was also unethical (Katz, 1992).

Today, researchers must abide by basic ethical norms when conducting research (Canadian Institutes of Health Research, Natural Sciences and Engineering Research Council of Canada & Social Sciences and Humanities Research Council of Canada [TCPS2], 2014). Most important, they must consider whether they might harm their human or animal subjects when conducting their research. It is crucial to ensure that both human and animal subjects are protected and respected throughout the entire research process (TCPS2, 2014).

Research with Human Subjects

Researchers must obtain informed consent from their subjects before beginning research. *Informed consent* means that subjects must know enough about the research to decide whether to participate, and they must agree to take part voluntarily. Furthermore, researchers have an ethical obligation to prevent both physical and mental harm to their subjects. If there is any risk of harm, they must warn subjects in advance. Researchers also must allow subjects to withdraw from a study at any time if they wish to stop participating. Finally, researchers have an obligation to protect the anonymity of their subjects.

Some psychological research cannot be done when subjects are fully informed about the purpose of the research, because people sometimes behave differently when under observation. To study people's normal behaviour, researchers sometimes have to deceive subjects. Deception is considered ethical only if the following apply:

- The study will give researchers some valuable insight.
- It would be impossible to do the study without deception.
- Subjects can learn the truth about the study's purpose and methods afterward.

Research with Animal Subjects

Although most psychological research involves human subjects, some professionals, such as psychologists, may also study animal subjects. Research with animal subjects has helped psychologists to do the following:

- Learn facts about animal species.
- Find ways to solve human problems employing animal models.
- Study questions that cannot be studied using human subjects for practical or ethical reasons.
- Refine theories about human behaviour.
- Improve human welfare.

Many people question the ethics of animal research because it can involve procedures such as deprivation, pain, surgery, and euthanasia. Psychologists have ethical obligations to treat animal subjects humanely and to perform research with animals only when the benefits of the research are clear.

People who are against animal research maintain three arguments:

1. Animals should have the same rights as humans.
2. Society should enact safeguards to protect the safety and welfare of animals.
3. Researchers should not put the well-being of humans above the well-being of animals.

REVIEW AND REFLECT

We have established that there are distinctly different routes to understanding the world of health and community practice using the qualitative, quantitative, and mixed-methods paradigms. It is important that we identify how these apparently opposing worldviews are applied to answer research questions that arise in practice. Within each paradigm, there are a number of approaches to research that are used to answer specific types of questions. These approaches to research are called *research methodologies*, a term we used in table 3.1. In addition to the philosophical and theoretical assumptions in research, research ethics is another fundamental element of research literacy. Through an understanding of basic principles of research ethics, you can more thoughtfully appraise the research for your practice. In chapters 6 and 7, you will explore in more depth specific research methodologies, the critical appraisal of these methodologies, as well as research ethics in qualitative and quantitative studies.

4 | HOW DO I SEARCH THE EVIDENCE FOR PRACTICE?

With contributions from Cari Merkley, Academic Librarian and Associate Professor, Mount Royal University, Calgary, Alberta

> "Knowledge is of two kinds. We know a subject ourselves, or we know where we can find information upon it."
>
> —Samuel Johnson

LEARNING OBJECTIVES

This chapter focuses on how to access and experience knowledge in a practical way. The goal is to give you the practical skills to embark on a literature review of a topic. You will be guided in general techniques for searching health and community practice library databases, keyword searching, referencing, organizing, and other information literacy skills—a must-have in this era of information overload. You will also be guided in some of the practical activities for writing a basic literature review for an assignment or report. After reading this chapter and completing the practical learning activities in appendix B, you will be able to do the following:

- Explain why you would conduct a literature review, as well as where and how to search for literature.
- Describe how to conduct and organize a search for efficiency and usefulness for practice.
- Describe why you would complete a literature review and how to go about doing so.

CHAPTER OUTLINE

- Why Does Searching Well Matter?
- What Is a Literature Review?
- Why Review the Literature?
- Defining Your Research Question
  - Tools to Help You Formulate Your Question
- Searching for Evidence
  - Peer-Reviewed Research
  - Finding Peer-Reviewed Research
  - Trade Publications
- Building a Search Strategy
- Evaluating Your Results
- How Do I Find Other Types of Resources?
  - Books
  - Popular Media Sources (Magazines and Newspapers)
  - Grey Literature
- General Web Searching Tips
- Keeping Track of What You Find and Citing Appropriately
- Reporting on Your Search: Annotated Bibliography and Literature Review
  - Annotated Bibliography
  - Literature Review
- Review and Reflect

WHY DOES SEARCHING WELL MATTER?

In an evidence-informed practice, there is an assumption that you are using the best available evidence, along with knowledge gained from your professional practice and your clients' individual needs, to guide your decisions. As a student or interprofessional practitioner, you will likely be required to conduct a literature review to find high-quality sources that will inform the arguments you are making in your assignments or practice. In health and community practice, all practitioners draw on what is already known in order to make choices in program design or to select individual or community interventions and so on. The pressing question to ask is, "How do you know if you have the best available evidence?" Searching in this context requires you to think carefully about balancing the need to be thorough with an understanding that searching for research literature is a time-consuming and iterative back-and-forth process.

This chapter takes you through the literature review process, first offering practical suggestions to make your searches efficient and effective, and then actually explaining how to write the literature review.

WHAT IS A LITERATURE REVIEW?

A *literature review* is an account of what has been published on a topic by accredited scholars and researchers. Occasionally, you will be asked to write a literature review as a separate assignment, but more often it is part of the introduction to an essay, report, project proposal, or thesis within a university or college setting or in your practice. In writing the literature review, your purpose is to convey to your reader what knowledge and ideas have been established on a topic, as well as the strengths and weaknesses of the concepts reviewed. As a piece of writing, the literature review must be defined by a guiding concept (e.g., your research objective or the problem or issue you are concerned with in practice). The stages of the literature review are as follows:

- Problem formulation—deciding the topic or field to be examined and its component issues or sub-topics
- Literature search—finding materials relevant to the topic being explored
- Data evaluation—determining which literature makes a significant contribution to the understanding of the topic
- Analysis and interpretation—discussing the findings and conclusions of pertinent literature in a formal scientific and structured manner, or informally (such as the analysis one might do for a university or college paper, proposal, or report)

WHY REVIEW THE LITERATURE?

You will review the literature for a variety of purposes. Perhaps the most important of these is to pull together what has been written on the problem area in order to highlight the significance or importance of the research. Health and community practitioners also review literature to inform their own understanding of the broad problem or issue, or to explain a question of concern in practice. Literature is also important in explaining and justifying the choices made in practice or for the pursuit of further knowledge. Understanding the literature review process is an important skill as a reader of research.

There are several steps to reviewing literature and different approaches to searching, recording, prioritizing, retrieving, reading, critiquing, and filing what you find. Let us begin by looking at a starting place to your search—defining the topic and questions you want to explore.

DEFINING YOUR RESEARCH QUESTION

Whether you are conducting your own research or looking for the research of others to use in an assignment or for practice, a well-defined research question is necessary (Fineout-Overholt & Johnston, 2005). How will you know if what you find is relevant if your question is unclear? Unclear questions also lead to more time spent searching and weeding through results. Searching, organizing, and reviewing the vast and growing body of literature are critical to almost every aspect of research literacy. Two main goals in the search: "(a) to retrieve only those papers that are relevant to the search question (this is called 'specificity'); and (b) not to miss any of those papers (this is called 'sensitivity')" (Kramer, 2010, p. 1).

The most common mistake novice researchers make is starting with a question that is too broad—for example, "What is the link between physical activity and health?" This is an important topic, but it is too big to do justice to in a single paper or study. A search for the terms *physical activity* and *health* in the research database PubMed finds over 90,000 individual documents that match these parameters. It is not feasible to read and assess how all of these items contribute to our understanding of the issue. Refining your research question will save considerable time and energy.

There are a number of ways to make your question more specific. Here are some questions to consider:

- Are you interested in a particular population? Factors such as age, gender, ethnic group, socioeconomic status, education levels, and pre-existing health conditions may play a role in whether the research you find is appropriate to apply to discussions around your population.
- What do all the terms in your question mean? For example, what do you mean by "health"? Are you interested in physical health or mental health? If you are interested in physical health, is there a particular measure of health that you would like to focus on (cardiovascular health, lower risk of chronic diseases, etc.)? Unpacking some of the concepts in your original question may help you narrow your focus.

- Does where the research was conducted matter? For example, would a research study looking at the effectiveness of a physical activity intervention that was conducted in Finland still be useful if the population you are working with is in Canada? Would research looking at the long-term mental health effects among Indigenous people who attended residential schools in Australia be relevant in the Canadian context? In many cases, the answer will be "yes." However, if your research is around a phenomenon specific to one country, you may want to specify the geographic region in your question.

Using the suggestions above, here is an example of a more specific and searchable research question: "Does practising yoga lead to decreased depressive symptoms?"

Tools to Help You Formulate Your Question

A number of tools have been developed to help students and practitioners create searchable and answerable research questions from problems or issues they encounter in their practice. The tools described below are not comprehensive. For an in-depth overview of the question formulation strategies available, please refer to the works of Kloda and Bartlett (2014), Melnyk and Fineout-Overholt (2015), or other research textbooks.

PICO—Patient Problem or Population, Intervention or Exposure, Comparison, Outcome

Patient problem or population, intervention or exposure, comparison, outcome (PICO) is one of the best-known tools for question formulation, emerging out of discussions around evidence-informed medicine (Richardson, Wilson, Nishikawa & Hayward, 1995). Later versions have added additional letters such as PICO(T), where T represents the timeframe in which an intervention is administered or an outcome measured (Melnyk & Fineout-Overholt, 2015). PICOT works with questions that are answerable with quantitative research (such as intervention, prognosis or prediction, diagnosis or diagnostic tests, etiology questions) and within qualitative research when asking a meaning question (Melnyk & Fineout-Overholt, 2015). Table 4.1 provides an example of a scenario translated into PICO format for a question best answered by a quantitative study. Table 4.2 offers an example of a scenario translated into a patient problem or population, issue of interest, outcome, and time (PIOT) format for a question best answered by a qualitative study.

Table 4.1: A Research Topic Scenario: PICO Format for a Quantitative Question

Scenario: A university student who is a long-term smoker is looking to quit. She has tried nicotine gum and patches in previous efforts to quit, and is wondering if using e-cigarettes might lead to more success.			
P (Patient Problem or Population)	**I** (Intervention or Issue of Interest)	**C** (Comparison Intervention or Issue of interest)*	**O** (Outcome)
University student who smokes	e-cigarettes	Other nicotine replacement therapies	Successful smoking cessation
Possible research question: Among young university students, does the use of e-cigarettes lead to greater levels of smoking cessation than other nicotine replacement therapies?			

Note: A comparison may not be identified in all questions.

Table 4.2: A Research Topic Scenario: PIOT Format for a Qualitative Question

Scenario: University student who smokes e-cigarettes wonders about the risk of getting lung cancer.			
P (Patient Problem or Population)	**I** (Issue of Interest)	**O** (Outcome)	**T** (Time)
University student who smokes	e-cigarettes	Risk of lung cancer	(not applicable)
Possible research question: How do university students who smoke e-cigarettes perceive their risk of lung cancer?			

COPES—Client-Orientated Practical Evidence Search

As the concept of evidence-informed practice has moved from medicine to other professions, PICOT has been adapted to reflect the concerns of researchers in those areas. Client-orientated practical evidence search (COPES) is a good example. According to Gibbs (2003), the COPES acronym is intended to remind practitioners in the helping professions that their research should be focused on the issues they encounter in their work and always relate back to the needs of their client or client group. COPES questions are similar to the PICOT framework in that they identify a population (referred to in this context as clients) as well as a problem, an action, a possible alternative, and outcome or what the professional hopes to accomplish (Gibbs, 2003). Table 4.3 provides an example of a structured COPES question.

Table 4.3: A Research Topic Scenario: COPES Format

Scenario: Caregivers of children with fetal alcohol spectrum disorder (FASD) wonder about the rewards of participating in different support programs.			
Client Group and Problem	**Action to Be Taken**	**Possible Alternative Course of Action***	**Preferred Outcome**
Caregivers of children with FASD	Participation in the step-by-step program	Participation in the coaching families program	Greater quality of life for families impacted by FASD
Possible research question: Among caregivers of children with fetal alcohol spectrum disorder, did participation in the step-by-step program lead to greater quality of life than for those who participated in the coaching families program?			

Note: An alternative course of action may not be identified in all questions. FASD = Fetal Alcohol Spectrum Disorder.
Source: Based on information from "The Effectiveness of a Community-Based Intervention for Parents with FASD," by K. Denys, C. Rasmussen & D. Henneveld, 2011, *Community Mental Health Journal, 47,* 209–219.

PS—Population, Situation

Another approach that may be useful is the population, situation (PS) format. PS asks you to identify the characteristics of the group you are interested in (i.e., the population or *P*), and what attitudes, beliefs, or experiences (i.e., the situation or *S*) you wish to explore among this group (Health Evidence, 2013). Table 4.4 offers an example of a PS format for a research topic.

Table 4.4: A Research Topic Scenario: PS Format

Scenario: School district leaders wonder about the values and views of high school students regarding new initiatives and clubs supporting gay–straight alliances.	
P **(Population)**	**S** **(Situation)**
High school students	Attitudes toward gay–straight alliances
Possible research question: What are the perceptions and views of a general population of high school students, including students who identify as LGBTQ, in school district X?	

Additional frameworks that may work well with qualitative research questions are Cooke, Smith & Booth's (2012) sample, phenomenon of interest, design, evaluation, research type (SPIDER) and Booth's (2006) setting, perspective, intervention, comparison, evaluation (SPICE).

SEARCHING FOR EVIDENCE

Once you have a clearly formulated question to explore, you will need to decide what type of information would best answer it, as well as what tool or tools you will use to find those resources. This is the next step in the evidence-informed decision-making process (see figure 4.1). Tips for finding peer-reviewed research, trade publications, popular media sources, books, and grey literature will be discussed below.

Searching, organizing, and reviewing the vast and growing body of literature are critical to almost every aspect of research literacy. As stated at the beginning of this chapter, and worth repeating here, these are the two main goals in your search: "(a) to retrieve only those papers that are relevant to the search question (this is called 'specificity'); and (b) not to miss any of those papers (this is called 'sensitivity')" (Kramer, 2010, p. 1).

Figure 4.1: The Search Step in the Evidence-Informed Decision-Making Process

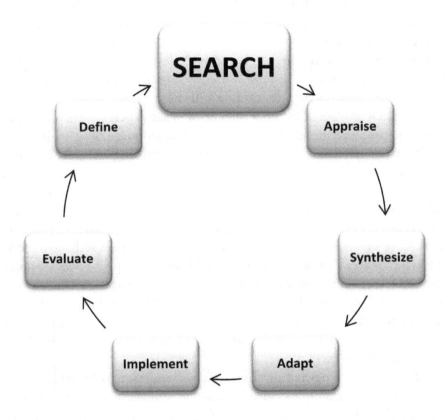

Source: Adapted from *Evidence-Informed Public Health*, by National Collaborating Centre for Methods and Tools, 2016, Hamilton, Canada: McMaster University. Copyright 2016 by McMaster University. Adapted with permission.

Peer-Reviewed Research

One of the key forms of evidence you will find in health and community studies is *peer-reviewed research*. Peer review, as a process, is intended to ensure only those studies with methods and findings that have been evaluated by other experts in the field and determined to be both original and of high quality are published. Peer-reviewed articles may also be described as "refereed" or "scholarly." Many journals use the double-blind form of peer review, in which the authors of the study and the reviewers are unaware of each other's identities, with the intention of preventing any personal bias from influencing the process.

As a general rule, peer-reviewed articles contain the following characteristics:

- Authors are clearly identified and their expertise supported by including the information of the universities or research organizations with which they are affiliated.
- Information is formally presented with few graphics beyond what is needed to present the data. Often research articles begin with an *abstract*, which provides an overview of the study.
- The article is written for an audience of other experts in the field and uses appropriate terminology and technical language.
- The paper includes considerable references to existing literature relevant to the study.

Unfortunately, most peer-reviewed journal articles are not labelled as such. In most cases, articles that match the characteristics described above would be peer-reviewed, but to be certain you may wish to visit the journal's website to confirm the editorial practices. Many search tools provide limits for peer-reviewed journals. In most cases, such limits are helpful but flawed, as the database includes all the content a journal may publish, including editorials or letters to the editor, which are typically not peer-reviewed. Use such limits, but evaluate each result against the criteria above to ensure what you are looking at would be considered a peer-reviewed research article.

Peer review is not a perfect process, so it is important to be critical of what you are reading. For example, flawed studies may make it to publication, only to be retracted later when issues with the research are revealed. One well-known example is an article authored by Dr. Andrew Wakefield et al. that appeared in the prominent British medical journal *The Lancet* in 1998. In the article, "Ileal-Lymphoid-Nodular Hyperplasia, Non-Specific Colitis, and Pervasive Developmental Disorder in Children," the authors suggested a potential link between the measles, mumps, and rubella (MMR) vaccine and the incidence of autism (Wakefield et al., 1998), which caught the media and public's attention when it was released and fuelled concerns around the potential adverse effects of vaccinations. However, no subsequent studies were able to support these results, and information emerged that the manner in which the study was conducted was misrepresented in the paper and did not meet ethical standards. As a result, the editors of *The Lancet* fully retracted the article from its publication record in 2010 ("Retraction," 2010). Even with such a prominent example of how the peer-review process failed to identify problems in a study before it was released, it continues to be held as a gold standard in quality control of published research.

Figure 4.2: How to Identify a Scholarly Article

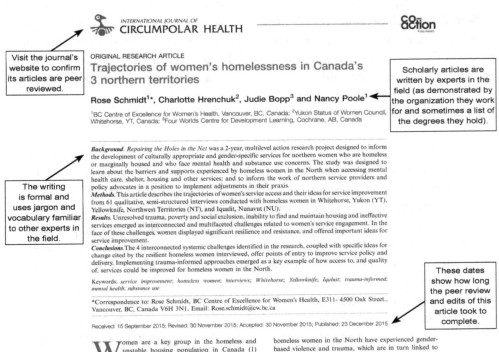

Visit the journal's website to confirm its articles are peer reviewed.

The writing is formal and uses jargon and vocabulary familiar to other experts in the field.

Scholarly articles are written by experts in the field (as demonstrated by the organization they work for and sometimes a list of the degrees they hold).

These dates show how long the peer review and edits of this article took to complete.

Most scholarly articles are very long because the author(s) have a lot of detail to share.

There will always be a long list of sources used in the article.

Source: Article screenshots taken from R. Schmidt, C. Hrenchuk, J. Bopp, & N. Poole (2015). Trajectories of women's homelessness in Canada's 3 northern territories. *International Journal of Circumpolar Health,* 74. Creative Commons Attribution 4.0 International License.

Finding Peer-Reviewed Research

There are many search engines and databases that will help you find peer-reviewed research on a topic. Some tools are freely available, while others require a subscription. Most university libraries subscribe to major databases in various fields of study for students and faculty to access. If you do not have access to databases at your workplace, most public libraries also have many of these databases.

Freely Available Tools

- PubMed (www.pubmed.gov) is the foremost database in the health sciences and is maintained by the United States National Library of Medicine. It contains over 25 million references to articles and books in the health sciences (United States National Library of Medicine, 2016). PubMed is the free version of Medline, which is a subscription database.
- Google Scholar (scholar.google.com) includes references to journal articles and books across disciplines. It is currently unknown how many documents are included in its search. One of the most useful features of Google Scholar is that it allows users to see who has cited a journal article since its publication. Other tools, such as Web of Science™ (Thomson Reuters, 2016) and Scopus (Elsevier, 2016), offer this function, but require a subscription to access. (see next section on Subscription Tools)

While both PubMed and Google Scholar are powerful free tools to help you identify what research has been published in a field, they do not provide full-text access to the articles themselves, unless the article has been made freely available by the journal publisher or author. Unfortunately, many of the articles published in health and community studies are within closed journals and require a paid subscription to access. Check with your university or your employer to see what subscriptions may be available to you.

Subscription Tools

Most research databases require an institutional subscription to access. Your university library, workplace, or professional association may provide this as part of your membership. While there may be overlapping content between these tools, they contain unique references or offer features specific to research in the discipline they support. As a result, most systematic searches of the literature will consult more than one database. Here are some examples of subscription databases in health and community studies:

- Medline—as mentioned above, Medline contains content that can also be found in PubMed.
- CINAHL—the Cumulative Index to Nursing and Allied Health Literature provides a much more focused search for those interested in nursing, midwifery, and allied health professions.
- PsycINFO—as the name suggests, PsycINFO focuses on the field of psychology, and would be of interest for research on topics relating to mental health, addiction, child development, and counselling.
- SocIndex—with broad coverage of sociology, SocIndex includes many social work journals.

To assist you with searching for answers to your questions, have a conversation with other professionals in your field or seek advice from a librarian who can provide you with suggestions for tools to use.

Trade Publications

Some of the databases listed above include professional newsletters or magazines aimed at specific professions, also known as trade publications. They resemble magazines in their layout and graphics. While such publications may occasionally include an article that has undergone peer review, most of the content is more conversational in tone, written by freelance writers who may not hold expertise in the subject matter, and only reviewed by the editor. Some examples of trade publications are *Canadian Nurse* and *Social Work Today*. These publications are useful windows into professional issues in your field, but are typically given less weight than peer-reviewed research. For a summary of the variety of scholarly publications you may search, refer to table 4.5.

BUILDING A SEARCH STRATEGY

Whether you are using a free tool like Google Scholar or a subscription database, it is important to consider the terms you use in your search carefully. If you have used PICOT or another tool to develop your research question, you have a logical start to the concepts you may wish to include as part of your search. It is not necessary to include all of the PICOT, COPE, or PS concepts you identified in your search. For example, you may only wish to include search terms relating to the intervention (*I*) and outcomes (*O*) you have identified in your PICOT framework. You might add additional information around your population (*P*) to further narrow your search results if your first attempt brings up too many sources.

Table 4.5: Types of Scholarly Publications

Type	Description
Research/Empirical	Papers reporting on the results of one or more studies or experiments, written by the individuals who conducted the research. This is considered one type of primary source. Look in the title or abstract for words like *study, research, measure, subjects, data, effects, survey,* or *statistical,* which might indicate empirical research.
Case study	Detailed account of clinically important cases of common and rare conditions.
Review	Summarizes the findings of other studies or experiments; attempts to identify trends or draw broader conclusions. Scholarly in nature but not a primary source or research paper; however, its references to other papers will include primary sources or research papers.
Systematic reviews	A systematic review is a summary of evidence on a particular research question that uses a rigorous process to identify, appraise, and synthesize studies to answer a question and come to a conclusion (Melnyk & Fineout-Overholt, 2015).
Meta-analysis	A meta-analysis is a specific kind of review paper—one with a mathematical synthesis of the results of two or more primary studies that addressed the same hypothesis in the same way.
Meta-synthesis	A meta-synthesis analyzes the findings for a research question from across the synthesis of qualitative studies (Melnyk & Fineout-Overholt, 2015).
Letters or communications	Short descriptions of important latest study or research findings, which are usually considered urgent for immediate publication. Examples: breakthroughs regarding cures or novel treatments, or a current outbreak of disease or social condition (e.g., addressing the traumatic stress response for refugees from a war zone).

(continued)

Table 4.5 (continued)

Theoretical	A paper containing or referring to a set of abstract principles related to a specific field of knowledge; characteristically it does not contain original empirical research or present experimental data, although it is scholarly.
Applied	Describes technique, workflow, management, or human resources issues.
Professional communications, book reviews, letters to the editor	Most scholarly journals publish papers that pertain to the workings of the profession but are not scholarly in nature.

Some general advice when conducting a search:

1. Consider synonyms for the concept for which you are searching. An article exploring the attitudes of a particular group of people might also describe them as beliefs, feelings, or opinions. You may wish to include all the synonyms in your search to ensure no articles are missed.

2. Consider replacing casual language with professional terminology (e.g., flu shot vs. influenza vaccine).

3. Spell out any acronyms (e.g., ADHD should be searched as "attention deficit and hyperactivity disorder") in order to find all of the relevant research.

4. Be aware of differences in Canadian, British, and American spelling practices. Many of the search tools are US-based, and dropping the "u" on words like "labour" can impact your search results.

5. Consider whether terminology in the field has changed over time. For example, many articles from the past would have used the term *sexually transmitted diseases*, rather than the current label *sexually transmitted infections*. If you would like to find all of the relevant articles, try using both terms.

6. Check the tool you are using for your search to see if it has subject headings or tags that it attaches to articles to describe them. For example, Medline and PubMed use *medical subject headings* (MeSH) as a way to describe an article and to group similar articles together.

If you use the subject heading in your search, you will find all of the articles that have been tagged with that term. Note that there can be a delay between an article being added to the database and it receiving its subject headings, so the most recent research may not yet be tagged. These subject headings, also known as controlled vocabulary, are often out of step with current usage, as they are infrequently updated. In some cases, you may even find the terminology used by the database to be offensive (e.g., while MeSH includes a heading for *Inuit*, the headings within the CINAHL database still use the term *Eskimo* to describe the same population). However, knowing how the database itself categorizes the information will be helpful to ensure that your search is thorough.

7. Many tools like Medline, PubMed, CINAHL, and PsycINFO have age limits that can be applied to your results to focus on studies that looked at a population within a particular age range. In many cases, it may be more effective to use these limits than to try to identify all the synonyms that may have been used to describe older adults or adolescents. Most databases have specific commands that can be incorporated into your search. For example, a very common command that works in almost all databases, as well as Google Scholar, is placing quotation marks around a phrase (e.g., "health promotion") to indicate that you wish to find results where these two words appear together in this exact order. Using the asterisk (*) will enable you to find various word forms (e.g., to search for all the possible endings to a word); for example, in some databases typing *canad** will find both *Canada* and *Canadian*. The symbol may vary depending on the database, so refer to the help section to confirm which commands work in the tool that you are using.

You should be aware that databases generally also use Boolean language (AND, OR, and NOT) to describe the relationships between different search terms. For example, "yoga AND depression" will only find results that contain both terms. On the other hand, "attitudes OR beliefs" will look for sources that use either term. Used less frequently, NOT is a way to exclude results containing a particular word. Increasingly, the basic search functions in most databases act much like Google, which automatically adds the word AND between any words typed. However, a thorough search may still require you to build your search, step by step, with the aid of the Boolean language. Table 4.6 provides examples of an advanced search in Medline in which each concept of the research question is searched separately using subject headings as well as keywords before being combined. In these examples, the *MH* in front of a term indicates that it is a MeSH subject heading.

Table 4.6: Advanced Search in Medline for the Research Question: Is Taking Vitamin C an Effective Treatment for the Common Cold?

Search 7 (S7)	S3 AND S6
Search 6 (S6)	S4 OR S5
Search 5 (S5)	"common cold"
Search 4 (S4)	(MH "rhinovirus") OR (MH "common cold")
Search 3 (S3)	S1 OR S2
Search 2 (S2)	"vitamin C"
Search 1 (S1)	(MH "ascorbic acid")

While you may not take the time to build such a search in every instance, taking a thorough approach to building your search is critical when you need to ensure that no sources are inadvertently missed. Keep an eye on your results—the titles of the articles you find may generate additional keywords that you may wish to go back and add to your search to make it more comprehensive.

EVALUATING YOUR RESULTS

Once you have a list of search results, it is important to evaluate them for their quality as well as how well they answer your research question. Evidence-informed practice in the health sciences often uses the evidence pyramid to help researchers and practitioners decide how different types of sources should be weighted in decision making. In the 6S pyramid model (see figure 4.3) proposed by DiCenso, Bayley, and Haines (2009), researchers are encouraged to use the highest level of evidence available to them in answering their question. Not every question will have evidence available at each level. All that might be available in an emerging field is an individual study reporting original research, the lowest level of evidence in the pyramid.

Systems, the highest level of evidence available in this model, refer to computerized decision support systems that incorporate the most up-to-date research (DiCenso et al., 2009). This level of evidence is very rare. More often, however, students and interprofessional practitioners in health and community studies may only go as far as the summaries layer which includes evidence-informed clinical practice guidelines. More information on how to locate summaries will be provided in the discussion on finding grey literature presented later in this chapter (see the Grey Literature section). Syntheses, which include systematic reviews, meta-analyses, and meta-syntheses, are often found in both free and subscription search tools. Organizations that are known for their creation of syntheses are the Cochrane Library (www.thecochranelibrary.com) and the Joanna Briggs Institute database (http://journals.lww.com/jbisrir/).

Figure 4.3: The 6S Pyramid

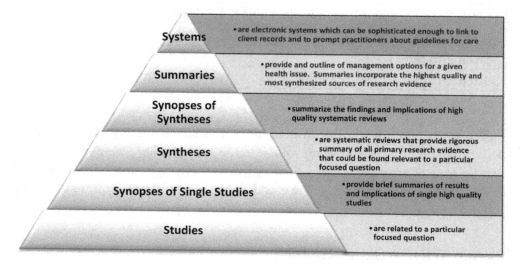

Systems • are electronic systems which can be sophisticated enough to link to client records and to prompt practitioners about guidelines for care

Summaries • provide and outline of management options for a given health issue. Summaries incorporate the highest quality and most synthesized sources of research evidence

Synopses of Syntheses • summarize the findings and implications of high quality systematic reviews

Syntheses • are systematic reviews that provide rigorous summary of all primary research evidence that could be found relevant to a particular focused question

Synopses of Single Studies • provide brief summaries of results and implications of single high quality studies

Studies • are related to a particular focused question

Source: Adapted from *Evidence-Informed Public Health*, by National Collaborating Centre for Methods and Tools, 2016, Hamilton, Canada: McMaster University. Available at: http://www. nccmt.ca/eiph/search-eng.html.

Most results found by the search tools used to locate peer-reviewed literature will fall into the bottom of the pyramid, with the already noted exception of systematic reviews and meta-analyses (syntheses) and critiques of individual studies that appear in journals such as *Evidence-Based Nursing* or *ACP Journal Club* (synopses of studies). Even at this level of the pyramid, however, there is an additional hierarchy of which individual study types are seen to yield the best evidence. For example, a randomized control trial is viewed to provide better evidence for a quantitative question than a cohort or case cohort study, and all three are seen to be superior to a single case study. Where qualitative research studies fall within this ranking system is still under debate. Daly et al. (2007) suggest that some of the reluctance to use qualitative research as evidence in practice is linked to researchers' uncertainty around how to evaluate its quality and apply it to practice. They propose privileging those more "generalizable" (Daly et al., 2007, p. 43) qualitative studies that provide thorough description of the theoretical underpinnings of the study, detail the process by which participants were selected and the data analyzed, and provide a rich detailed reporting of results. On the other hand, Trochim (2016) states, "To say that one or the other approach is 'better' is a trivializing of a far more complex topic than a dichotomous choice" (para. 1). Trochim (2016) asserts that there is merit in combining quantitative and qualitative methods, referred to as "'mixed methods' approach" (para. 1) in answering certain questions. If you are interested in reading more about the qualitative versus quantitative research approaches, refer to other research textbooks where this debate is addressed (for instance, in Creswell, 2014).

Regardless of where the study falls in the hierarchy, it is important to assess its quality against the ideals for its study type and its potential applicability to your research question. There are many tools available to assist you in this critical appraisal, including chapters 5, 6, and 7 in this textbook. Additional recommended reading is Greenhalgh's *How to Read a Paper: The Basics of Evidence-Based Practice* (2014), a classic text in evidence-informed practice now in its fifth edition.

HOW DO I FIND OTHER TYPES OF RESOURCES?

There are many other types of information resources that are not always captured in databases or search engines. Here are some of the most common types of information you may find yourself searching for and some tips for their retrieval.

Books
Books in health and community studies can provide a distilled version of existing practice-related research, explore important theory in depth, walk you through particular skills, or take readers through the history of the profession. Due to the considerable time lag between the writing and the publication of books, there are often concerns about the currency and accuracy of the research presented and they may not be included in research syntheses. Also, not all books take a scholarly approach to their subject matter; consider carefully the fit between the authors' backgrounds and the subject they examine, as well as how they have documented their sources for the information presented. Each library has a searchable listing of the books in their collection (known as the library catalogue). You can also use WorldCat® (www.WorldCat.org) to search across individual library catalogues to find a library near you that holds the book you need.

Popular Media Sources (Magazines and Newspapers)

Magazines and newspapers provide a window into current events and popular opinion. As they are competing with each other for the public's dollar, more attention is paid to graphics and headlines to entice readers. The articles they produce are much easier to read than scholarly articles and tend not to use much technical or specialist language. Quality control of articles, in this context, may consist of fact checking and editorial review, but not a peer review. It is important, however, not to dismiss magazines and newspapers when researching. In some cases, they may be the only sources available for information on emerging or local news. They provide a useful example of how social issues are framed for the public and the public's reaction to them. As students and professionals, it is also important to acknowledge that for many members of the public, their understanding of health or social issues may be drawn from these sources, because they are far more accessible in print or electronic form than more academic materials, which may be written or priced out of their reach. These sources will enable you to be aware of what the public is reading so that you can bring other more reliable sources in to either confirm or counteract some of the information presented.

Grey Literature

Grey literature is material produced by governments, associations, non-profit organizations, universities, and other institutions as they go about their business. What separates grey literature from other publications is that publishing is not the main focus of the organizations that produce the material (Farace & Schöpfel, 2010). Most grey literature does not undergo the formal peer-review process used by journals, but they still may be informed and reviewed by other professionals in the course of their production. Examples of grey literature include clinical practice guidelines, government documents, dissertations and theses, professional association documents, and statistics.

Searching for grey literature is complicated by the fact that there is no single comprehensive listing of these works and no one place to find them. Often a pointed search of an organization's website is the best option available. Libraries currently do not make it their practice to collect all these works, so they can appear and disappear online unexpectedly. It is a good idea to save copies of those documents you may need to refer to again in the future, rather than relying on a weblink to remain active indefinitely.

Grey literature must also be evaluated. For government, agency, or think tank reports as well as white papers, using the currency, reliability, authority, accuracy, and purpose (CRAAP) test, developed for websites, can be helpful.

- **Currency:** Not always an issue for a document, but make sure it is dated and you have accessed the most recent version.
- **Reliability:** Does the author provide supporting references? Do the sources have active links?
- **Authority of author or organization:** What is the mission of the organization? What type of organization is it?
- **Accuracy:** Does the content demonstrate reliability, truthfulness, and correctness?
- **Purpose or point of view:** Is there a bias? Is the purpose clear? Are outcomes of the report supported?

If you seek further resources, many helpful CRAAP charts for evaluating sources can be readily found on the Internet.

Practice Guidelines

The Health and Medical Division of the US National Academies of Sciences, Engineering, and Medicine (formerly, the Institute of Medicine) defines *clinical practice guidelines* as "statements that include recommendations intended to optimize patient care that are informed by a systematic review of evidence and an assessment of the benefits and harms of alternative care options" (Institute of Medicine, 2011, p. 1). It is the use of evidence and its rigorous critique by practising professionals that help to place practice guidelines in the *Summaries* layer of the 6S evidence pyramid (see figure 4.3). Practice guidelines can be found for health professionals in many fields including medicine, nursing, public health, speech language pathology, and midwifery. Some practice guidelines may be published in journals sponsored by professional associations, but others will only be published online. There are a few websites that attempt to pull together guidelines from various sources including the *National Guideline Clearinghouse* (Agency for Healthcare Research and Quality, n.d.) and the Canadian Medical Association's (2016) *Canadian Practice Guidelines Infobase*. Another free tool, the Trip Database (2016), also includes links to practice guidelines in its search results.

Government Documents

All levels of government (municipal, provincial, and federal) produce documents of interest to researchers. The volume and range of publications is overwhelming—legislation, records of debates in Parliament, departmental annual reports, information for citizens, and more. Most university libraries, recognizing the complexity of this information, have created guides to help users navigate these resources. Ask your librarian for suggestions.

Often, the search functions of individual department websites are less effective than using a targeted Google search (www.google.com). For example, adding "site:gc.ca" after your keywords in a Google search will only return results from websites hosted by the Canadian federal government (e.g., "supervised injection site:gc.ca").

Dissertations and Theses

Dissertations and theses, produced in the course of doctoral and masters' level graduate work in universities, are in-depth investigations of research questions. In many cases, these works will be adapted and published as scholarly articles or books at a later date. Once difficult to access given their limited print circulation, dissertations and theses are increasingly made available electronically either through free collections like the Theses Canada Portal (Library and Archives Canada, 2016) or subscription resources like ProQuest Dissertations and Theses Global (ProQuest, n.d.).

Professional Association Publications

Professional associations are prolific producers of documents. Codes of ethics, position statements, and commissioned research may all be featured on an association's website for the public to view. In some cases, access to documents may be limited to members. In such circumstances, consider contacting the association for assistance if you are not a member.

Statistics

Researchers will encounter statistics in both peer-reviewed and grey literature. Statistics are collected by researchers, government agencies, intergovernmental institutions like the United Nations, as well as non-profit organizations. Much like grey literature as a whole, statistics can be difficult to locate, and the quality of the data should always be carefully scrutinized. One strategy for locating statistics is to identify organizations that would be interested in collecting data on your topic and to explore their websites carefully. It may also be useful to consider how the data could be collected, such as counting users of particular services or surveys. Whenever possible, it is better to go to the originator of statistical data, rather than relying on numbers reported in the popular media, as statistics and the information they convey rely heavily on how they are framed.

GENERAL WEB SEARCHING TIPS

When most people think of searching the web, their first stop is Google (www.google.com). There is no denying that Google has become the dominant search engine, but it is important to remember that, like any tool, the way results are presented is not necessarily objective. Many quality resources do not make it onto the first page of results. Google states that the number of times someone has linked to the site and how recently it has been updated factor into rankings, but other factors in the algorithm are not known publicly (Google, n.d.). As mentioned above, it is possible to limit your search results to a particular web domain (e.g., include "site:gc.ca" in your search parameters to limit results to Canadian federal government websites). Another helpful domain you might limit your results to is .edu (e.g., include "site:edu" in your search parameters), which will bring back results from American colleges and universities. Your search is also coloured by where it is conducted; Google presents results that are assumed to be more relevant to your geographic location (e.g., privileging Canadian and American websites). If you are interested in sources from other countries, searching that country's specific Google page may be more productive, such as searching www.google.com.au for documents specific to Australia (Bonato, 2013).

KEEPING TRACK OF WHAT YOU FIND AND CITING APPROPRIATELY

It is essential that you find a way to organize your resources so that when it comes time to begin writing, the information you need is at your fingertips. Whether it is index cards, a Microsoft Word document, or a free reference management tool like Mendeley (2016) or Zotero (Center for History and New Media, 2016), find a system that works for you. You may also find it helpful to keep track of the terms you used in your searches, in case you need to go back and revisit or rerun any of those searches in the future. Most tools will allow you to save or print out your strategy for future use.

Make sure you give credit to the originators of any ideas you include in your work by citing them appropriately. Plagiarism—the use of others' work without proper attribution—is unethical and a violation of codes of conduct that govern universities. Plagiarism may be accidental (e.g., you copy a phrase into your document from the web and later forget that the words used were not your own), but this is still considered plagiarism and is subject to academic sanctions. Always enclose any phrases that are not your own in quotation marks and provide information about the source, using the appropriate citation style for your field of study, such as the American Psychological Association (APA) publication format (American Psychological Association, 2010). If you are using an idea and describing it in your own words (i.e., paraphrasing), you need to ensure that you have changed not only the words, but also the order in which the words are presented and structured. Even when paraphrasing, you must cite the source (i.e., credit the person who first presented that idea or concept). There are many free guides about citation on the Internet. We recommend that you refer to those produced by educational institutions to ensure that they are of higher quality (e.g., The Purdue Online Writing Lab [OWL], National Research Council Purdue University, The Writing Lab, 2016). Furthermore, there is room for interpretation in how citation styles are applied, so if your university has produced its own guide for students, it is best to follow that documentation so that you can be sure you and your instructor are using the same frame of reference.

REPORTING ON YOUR SEARCH: ANNOTATED BIBLIOGRAPHY AND LITERATURE REVIEW

A summary of citations (annotated bibliography) and formal literature review are two of the more common ways you will report on your search. Sometimes people confuse literature reviews with annotated bibliographies; they are quite different in format, although they are similar in purpose in that both present a survey of the literature.

Annotated Bibliography

An annotated bibliography is a list of citations to books, articles, and documents. Each citation is followed by a brief (usually 150 words in length) descriptive and evaluative paragraph (i.e., the annotation). The purpose of the annotation is to inform the reader of the relevance, accuracy, and quality of the sources cited. To write a good annotated bibliography, you need to be concise, evaluative, critical, and comparative:

- Concise: Get to the point of what the book or article is about in few words—summarize.
- Evaluative: Determine who the author is, what his or her expertise is in the topic, how reliable the information is.
- Critical: Reflect on the strengths and weaknesses of the work. Ask yourself, "What is missing?"
- Comparative: Describe how the book or article compares to other similar works.

In assessing each piece, consideration should be given to a general level of appraisal or critique. Chapter 5 provides more detailed levels of appraisal for the different kinds of research papers you will read. A brief or general level of appraisal, however, involves review of the following aspects of the papers you are reading:

- Credibility: What are the author's credentials? Are the author's arguments supported by evidence (e.g., primary historical material, case studies, narratives, statistics, or recent scientific findings)?
- Objectivity: Is the author's perspective balanced or prejudicial? Is contrary data considered, or is certain information ignored so as not to disprove the author's point?

- Persuasiveness: Which of the author's theses are the most or least convincing?
- Value: Are the author's arguments and conclusions convincing? Does the paper ultimately contribute in any significant way to an understanding of the subject? Is the article useful for health and community practice?

Literature Review

As previously noted, writing an annotated bibliography is a different task from composing a literature review. In a literature review, you will provide an overview of the subject, issue, or topic under consideration. The general format is an exploration of a variety of current and classic research papers on a topic: those in support of a particular position, those against, and those offering entirely different perspectives. The review provides an explanation of how each work is similar to and how it varies from the others. Finally, a basic literature review will draw conclusions as to which arguments are most convincing and where there remain questions about the topic.

What Kinds of Literature Reviews Are Written?

Some forms of literature review (systematic review, meta-analysis, and meta-synthesis) are formal research studies in and of themselves. *Systematic reviews* "use a specific procedure to search the research literature, select the studies to include in their review, and critically evaluate the studies they find" (Nelson, 2013, p. 139). In a *meta-analysis*, the researcher reviews research findings in a quantitative approach "by transforming the data from individual studies into what is called an *effect size* and then pooling and analyzing this information. The basic goal in meta-analysis is to explain why different outcomes have occurred in different studies" (Roberts & Ilardi, 2003, p. 197). Finally, a *meta-synthesis* is a type of "qualitative study that uses as data the findings from other qualitative studies linked by the same or related topic" (Zimmer, 2006, p. 312).

For the kinds of literature reviews required for students and interprofessional practitioners when doing assignments, proposals, or reports in practice, the formal and systematic structures of a systematic review, meta-analysis, or meta-synthesis are not expected. You will most likely undertake a more general format—often just a few paragraphs or pages of summary, synthesis, and analysis. The literature review is a way of demonstrating two things:

1. The literature search—you have found the materials needed to provide background and current thinking about your topic.
2. Your understanding and analysis—you have put what you found from your search into the context of your project, report, or question.

You may be wondering how many sources you need to conduct a literature review. Unfortunately, there is no magic number for how many sources you are going to need for your literature review. It all depends on the topic and what type of literature review you are doing:

- Are you working on an emerging topic? If so, you will not find many sources, which is good because you are trying to prove that this is a topic that needs more research.
- Are you working on a mature topic, something that has been studied extensively? Then you are going to find many sources and you will want to limit how far you want to look back (e.g., limit your search to just the last 10 years instead of 50). The limits and constraints you place on retrieving sources will depend on the topic.
- Always consult assignment or proposal guidelines to ensure you meet the specified criteria.

How Do I Write a Literature Review for an Assignment, Proposal, or Report?

In your literature review, you will want to summarize major contributions of significant studies and articles to the body of knowledge under review, maintaining the focus established in the introduction. You will also evaluate the current stage of development for the body of knowledge reviewed, pointing out major methodological flaws or gaps in research, inconsistencies in theory and findings, and areas or issues pertinent to future study. Finally, you will conclude by providing some insight into the relationship between the central topic of the literature review and a larger area of study for health and community practice.

One common way to approach the presentation of a literature review is to start out broad and then become more specific. Think of it as continuum of what is known in relation to your topic or question. First, briefly explain the broad issues related to your questions or topic; you do not need to write much about this—just demonstrate that you are aware of the breadth of your subject. Then narrow your focus to deal with the studies that overlap with your topic and the studies that directly relate to your topic (see figure 4.4).

Ways to organize your literature review include the following:

- Chronological order of research papers and discoveries
- General to specific knowledge and discoveries
- Contrast or comparison of different findings
- Identification of overall trends
- Methodological focus or organized by the methods of study

- Development of knowledge in areas of problem, cause, and solution identification
- Topical order (or how topical and how many results you found in certain areas of the literature)

Figure 4.4: Presenting the Literature Review as a Continuum of Knowledge

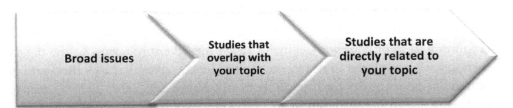

Literature reviews are usually written in third person. The first paragraph should be a road map of the rest of the literature review; for instance, it will describe the overall discoveries and how you are going to present what you found in your search and review. When presenting others' research, be clear about the assertions of the researchers, what their conclusions were, whether or not those conclusions were supported by the data. Be careful to synthesize rather than directly quote sentence after sentence. Finally, use signposts, headings, and transitions to clarify and summarize your discoveries in the literature. See box 4.1 for more specific writing tips.

Box 4.1: Writing Tips for Your Literature Review

- Do not over-quote. If you only quote from every single author you found, then you are not showing any original thinking or analysis. Instead use paraphrasing to report, in your own words, what the author was reporting or theorizing.
- Summarize findings, important sections, or a whole article—this is different from paraphrasing since you are not restating the author's words, but identifying the main points of what you are reading in a concise manner for your readers.
- When synthesizing your findings for the literature review (this is when you make comparisons, establish relationships between authors' works, point out weaknesses, strengths, and gaps), you still need to give credit to these sources.

The key elements of a basic literature review include providing an overview and argument, reading critically, writing analytically, and identifying areas for further research. This analytical way of writing asks that you try to summarize the arguments of different authors in relation to your own question or topic. Can you compare or contrast different authors' concepts or theories, or identify any emerging themes? You will need to present an argument or a series of points—do not just describe what different authors have written. Often you will find that your topic overlaps different subject disciplines, bringing in multiple perspectives and different sets of literature. Pointing this out and discussing it emphasizes the thoroughness of your work. Finally, relate the literature review to the bigger questions being explored in the topic. Try to identify areas that lack literature or research as opportunities for gaps to be filled (Wakefield, 2014; 2015). Refer to the chapter 4 learning activities in appendix B for a sample.

REVIEW AND REFLECT

Reviewing the research and known literature on a topic or question is a key skill in research literacy. It begins with searching the literature and builds to a review so that what is known, and where there are gaps in the research, can become clearer. Remember searching for evidence rarely progresses in a straight line. You may start with a research question, only to go back and modify it based on initial search results. You may identify additional search terms as you begin reading the articles you uncover and then need to go back to the databases to try them. This is completely natural, and giving yourself enough time to allow for these stops and starts may lessen the anxiety you feel about the process. It is also important to remember that you are not alone in this work. Fellow students, your instructor, or colleagues may be able to offer advice based on their own experiences. There is also a group of people for whom such searching of the literature is their area of expertise—librarians and other information specialists. Take advantage of the services your college, university, hospital, or local public library may offer. If you are feeling stuck in an endless maze of sources, sometimes a quick chat with a librarian can help redirect your search and get you back on track.

Writing up the literature review is a fairly standardized practice, and reading other reviews can help you learn how to write them. More than a descriptive account, a literature review requires that you write analytically. As a result, building on your research appraisal skills will strengthen the analysis in your literature reviews.

5 | HOW DO I APPROACH THE APPRAISAL OF A RESEARCH PAPER?

"I know the strengths and weaknesses of my teammates. I make my passing decisions accordingly."

—Steve Nash

LEARNING OBJECTIVES

This chapter focuses on how you will critically appraise research papers. The general anatomy of a research paper is discussed, as are generic steps of writing a research critique. After reading the chapter and completing the practical learning activities in appendix B, you will be able to do the following:

- Describe why research is critiqued.
- Describe the structure of a research paper.
- Explain the steps for critically appraising a research paper.
- Describe how to write a research critique.

CHAPTER OUTLINE

- Why Critique Research?
- What Is the General Structure of a Research Paper?
- What Are the Steps of Critical Appraisal of Research Papers?
  - Appraising the Source
  - Appraising the Literature Review
  - Appraising the Research Question
  - Appraising the Data
  - Appraising the Methods and Results—What Did They Do and What Did They Find?
  - Appraising the Conclusions
- How Do I Write a Research Critique?
- Review and Reflect

WHY CRITIQUE RESEARCH?

Critiquing what you find concerns the analysis of what is available, weighing the evidence, and determining the next best questions, gaps, and applications. The ability to critique requires the developed intellectual skills of critical thinking and appraisal. A thoughtful critique is aimed at the product of research—the research paper—not the researcher. A critique of a research paper involves a systematic and unbiased approach in order to determine the credibility and integrity of a study. Careful examination of all aspects of the research study is required in order to judge the meaning and significance of the research. Appraisal is an important step in the evidence-informed decision-making process (see figure 5.1). As Steve Nash would say, knowing the strengths and weaknesses of the studies you are reading, you can make your decisions accordingly.

All studies have limitations, which can potentially lead to problems of inaccuracies in data and outcomes of analysis, or limitation in application of those findings to different practice environments. An ability to recognize both the strengths and limitations of the research is essential. Generally, appraisal of a research paper is done to broaden understanding and to summarize what is known as a means of decision making for practice or as a base for the conduct of a new research study (Burns & Grove, 2011).

Figure 5.1: The Appraisal Step in the Evidence-Informed Decision-Making Process

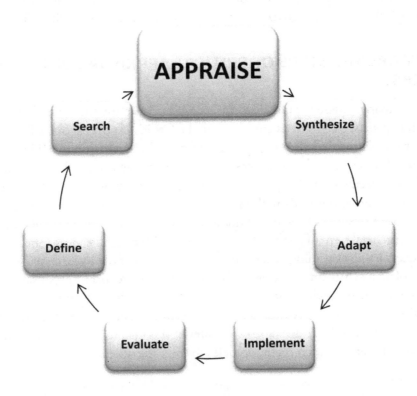

Source: Adapted from *Evidence-Informed Public Health,* by National Collaborating Centre for Methods and Tools, 2016, Hamilton, Canada: McMaster University.

WHAT IS THE GENERAL STRUCTURE OF A RESEARCH PAPER?

As introduced in chapter 1, a research paper is an article written by authors who have either collected and analyzed their own data (primary data analysis) or analyzed data that has been collected by someone else (secondary data analysis). Regardless, a research paper should consist of new, original work that has not been presented before. It is not simply a summary of research that others have done; rather, it is the presentation of new analyses. In a research paper, the authors generally begin their report with a literature review, or a summary and synthesis of information on similar research on the topic. Characteristically, a research paper explains why the current paper is important, describes the data and methods used in the research, presents findings, and discusses the results, limitations, and implications of the study. In short, a research paper generally contains the following sections: abstract, introduction (including the literature review), methods (including the methodology, ethics, sample, data, and analysis), results, and discussion (including limitations, implications, and conclusions) (American Psychological Association, 2010). The purpose of each section is outlined in table 5.1.

WHAT ARE THE STEPS OF CRITICAL APPRAISAL OF RESEARCH PAPERS?

There are many different guidelines and tools available for the *critical appraisal* of research papers (see collections compiled by the Critical Appraisal Skills Programme, 2013, or the National Collaborating Centre for Methods and Tools, 2011). There are also many distinct research approaches that will adjust how you conduct your appraisal or critique. Specific critical appraisal or qualitative research is discussed in chapter 6, with quantitative and mixed-methods research addressed in chapter 7. Here you will be introduced to some of the broad questions to ask yourself as you read, and to the beginning general steps of appraisal, which begins with critical reading (Spears, 2013). The process involves reading and reviewing the sources of the research paper, and, in the case of an assignment or review of the literature for a report or proposal, writing a discussion of the research available and strengths and limitations of the results. Some broad tips for starting the critical appraisal process are found in box 5.1. The steps in the process are introduced in more detail later in this chapter, with specific questions to ask for different research methodologies in the subsequent chapters.

Box 5.1: Tips for Conducting a Research Appraisal

- Read and critique the entire study.
- Examine the previous research and expertise of the authors.
- Examine the organization and presentation of the research report.
- Identify the strengths and weaknesses of the study.
- Be objective and realistic in identifying the study's strengths and weaknesses based on standards related to the research methodology (qualitative, quantitative, or mixed methods).
- Identify relevancy for application or gaps with suggestions for future studies.

Source: Adapted from *Understanding Nursing Research* (5th ed.), by N. Burns & S. Grove, 2011, Toronto, Canada: W.B. Saunders. Reprinted with permission.

Table 5.1: Anatomy of a Research Paper

Section	Function	Your Reading and Use
Abstract	Brief summary of the research including the main questions, methods, results, and implications.	Provides a general sense of the research paper. Briefly shows if this is what you are looking for to respond to your question or problem in practice. The abstract will give you a good idea of what to expect from the piece as a whole (including topic or purpose, questions or hypotheses, main results, and implications).
Introduction	Introduces the topic of interest, the purpose of the study, and provides background research leading to the new questions explored in the study.	Connects you to how others may be thinking of the topic. Shows sources of related research that may address the questions at hand.
Methods	Describes the mechanics of the study, including participants, measures used, and procedure.	Understand the design of the study and the tools used to experiment or explore the topic in a systematic way.
Results	Describes what was found in the study, highlighting the numbers (statistics) with tables and narrative description, or narrative analysis of textual or visual data excerpts.	Begin to see and know what was found in the research study.
Discussion	Describes the limitations and implications of the study.	Understand how these findings relate to your practice and whether changes in your practice are advisable.

Appraising the Source

In this first level of appraisal, you ask yourself exactly what it is that you are reading. The first thing to examine when reading a research article is where the article was found. Is it from a peer-reviewed journal? Was it published on the Internet? Who is the author? Is it from a government or professional practice source? Typically, peer-reviewed journal articles are considered to be the highest quality, because they have undergone a rigorous review process prior to publication. Most academic journals are peer-reviewed, while many research briefs and reports found on the Internet are not (see chapter 4 for more information on searching for sources). Also consider the specific source of the authors of the research. What are their credentials? Do they have other research on the topic cited? Do they have an affiliation that makes them biased for any reason (e.g., are they employed or based at a firm or company with an agenda or specific interest in the topic)? Are any author biases declared up front? Do the sponsors or funders of the research pose a conflict of interest in some way (e.g., a research study on the efficacy of a herbal sleep aid is funded by the producer of the product)?

As you review these questions about the source of the research, be careful not to let judgments about where the research paper is published or who wrote it dominate your appraisal of the trustworthiness and relevance (Critical Appraisal Skills Programme, 2013). Source appraisal is just one element of the research paper you will review to determine the strengths and limitations of the research. Using critical appraisal skills and tools enables users of research evidence to reach their own judgments. You will want to include these specific questions in your appraisal of the source:

- Where and when was the article published?
- Who wrote the article?
- Does the source reflect the genre of the source's discipline (or disciplines)?
- Does the source offer sufficient detail? Are there gaps in the description or places with unnecessary description?
- Does the source present the information logically?
- Does the source present an objective viewpoint? Does the author seem to have a bias or blind spot?

Appraising the Literature Review

All research papers begin with a review of the other research that has taken place on this topic. A good literature review should do the following:

- Describe research findings from a variety of researchers, over time, and in broad and specific relation to the topic.
- Concentrate on research papers from peer-reviewed journals.

This is not merely a list or annotation of all the known research on the topic but should summarize and synthesize the existing knowledge. As discussed in chapter 4, the overall goal of the literature review is to provide an integrative summary of other research findings and the questions that remain unanswered or require additional research. In your appraisal, you will want to look at the depth, breadth, and currency of the literature reviewed. Are there any obvious omissions (e.g., has literature that refutes one perspective or another been left out)? Again, there is no fixed number of research papers that should be in a literature review, and if the topic is novel and unexplored there may be little by way of research available for review. Your intent in this process is to appraise for the quality and quantity of the review, as it sets up the research process.

Appraising the Research Question

In your appraisal of the research question, you are asking questions about the goals, value, and purpose of the study. Authors will often follow the literature review by identifying their research question and how their study fits into the existing knowledge base. It should not simply replicate what other researchers have done before, but instead must offer something new. In your appraisal, you will assess the value and need for the research. You should also appraise what the authors propose as a research question (Dunifon, 2005). Frequently, authors will state the research question as a hypothesis by offering a prediction of what they think they will find, and will test that hypothesis to see if it holds true (e.g., "Children who have less screen time will have higher test scores"). However, many times authors will simply state the general question they seek to answer without offering a hypothesis (e.g., "Is screen time associated with test scores?"). In some studies, there is no hypothesis and the question should explain the kind of inquiry being conducted (e.g., an exploratory inquiry). A study exploring the screen time experiences of children or families would not have a hypothesis, but the issue and question should still be stated (e.g., "What are the experiences of children and families regarding the use of screen time?"). Regardless of the study purpose or methodology, you will want to ask the following questions in your appraisal of the question and purpose:

- Is the research question stated up front, and is the question answered by the end of the research paper?
- Is the research problem significant and important for health and community practice?
- What was the purpose of the study?

Appraising the Data

When appraising the data, you will review the participants or subjects in the study and the data being collected. Research papers should provide a good description of the data collected and used in the analysis. One important aspect of the data that requires consideration is the sample or chosen participants for the study. In your appraisal, make note of the sample size and the appropriateness of the choice of sample for the question being asked.

In terms of the sample size, researchers must choose between obtaining less detail on a large number of people and obtaining more detail on a small number of people. Practical realities, the design of the study, and the questions asked in the study will all dictate the appropriate sample size. There are no absolute standards for the ideal number of subjects in a study, but keep in mind that there are always trade-offs in terms of sample size. For instance, the smaller the sample size, the more difficult it will be to conduct statistical analyses and the less reliable and generalizable these analyses will be. Smaller sample sizes, however, are desired in qualitative studies, where the focus is on representativeness and believability rather than generalizability. Representativeness means that the data should reflect the individuals whom the authors hope to represent or describe in their sample (Dunifon, 2005). For example, a sample could represent the stories of families in a specific community recreation program, or the experiences of seniors who are homeless in Vancouver.

Appraising the Methods and Results—What Did They Do and What Did They Find?

As explained in chapter 3, there are several types of research methods that researchers may use (e.g., surveys, interviews, observations, etc.). These methods and the specific ways of appraising their use and analysis of data will be elaborated on in the following two chapters.

As a broad appraisal, however, you can review whether the methods chosen were the best fit to respond to the overarching research question. In this appraisal, your critical thinking is the best guide. For example, in a study addressing individual experiences and outcomes of a standing desk intervention, you might question the use of a group interview method. For assessing individual experiences, one-on-one interviews may be a more appropriate strategy for data gathering.

You will also want to appraise the specific research measures or instruments selected in the study. The authors should tell you how each variable used in their analyses was measured and defined. For example, if the authors are measuring the effect of screen time on test scores, how are both screen time and test scores defined? Are they using a widely used scale? Are they using several items or a single item? Did they create their own measure, and if so, how did they do it? These questions are further explained in chapter 7.

When deciding how to measure data, such as test scores, researchers can either use assessments that have already been developed and tested by others, or they can create their own measures. If they use an assessment that has already been developed and tested, the authors will typically cite the fact that it is widely used and has been shown to measure what it really claims to be measuring (referred to as *validity*). If researchers create their own measure, they need to prove that their instrument actually measures what they say it does (Creswell, 2014). Frequently, they do this by (a) comparing the chosen measure to others that are already proven to be valid to show that the two measures are capturing similar phenomena; or (b) running a pilot test of the measure and checking the results before proceeding to the main study.

As you are reading and appraising the methods, analysis, and results, do not worry if you are unable to make complete sense of all the analysis and tables. Like with learning any language, this is knowledge that will develop with use. The specific details and terminology will be elaborated on in the following chapters focused on the appraisal of qualitative, quantitative, and mixed-methods research papers. The goal as a beginning critical reviewer of research is to gain a basic understanding of what the researchers did, and then, by reading the text and tables, evaluating how believable their main findings were and if the claims they made are realistic or being oversold. Table 5.2 illustrates a critical reading of research results and asks the question, "Has the author overgeneralized the research results?"

You will want to ask these specific questions in your appraisal about the research design, methodology, and methods:

- What is the analytical approach or theoretical framework (e.g., a feminist analysis, a critical analysis, an application of a specific theoretical model)?
- What was the methodology for the study (e.g., a case study, ethnography, a content analysis, or an experimental study)?
- Does the methodology reflect or augment other studies of the same topic?
- What makes this method feasible? How realistic is it?
- Why will this method produce data that will answer the research question?

- How does the method address questions of validity?
- Was the research conducted ethically and following *Tri-Council Policy Statement* (TCPS2, 2014) guidelines?

Table 5.2: Critical Appraisal of Results: A Research Study Example

Appraisal question: Has the author overgeneralized the results in the paper?	
Research Paper Excerpt: "Collaborative community refugee response: Exploring the way forward"	**Critical Reading and Appraisal**
Each group interview, comprised of government, non-governmental, and for-profit refugee service providers (n = 10), was tape recorded and took between 60 and 90 minutes to complete. Recordings of the interviews were listened to and transcribed. During this period, hunches or working hypotheses were identified, which were explored in subsequent individual interviews. The major theme of "fulfilling our mandates—together but separately" was identified as providing insight into how service providers view "community collaboration."	The author has used the findings from a very small sample size that may not represent a sufficient range of perspectives to support a major line of argument about how community groups view collaboration.
The remainder of this paper will focus on an exploration of this theme and its significant implications for community health and services.	The author infer that the results gained from interviewing these community service providers can be generalized to all communities.

Appraising the Conclusions

In appraising the conclusions, you ask yourself: So what? What does it all mean? At the end of the paper, the authors should summarize what they found and tie their results in with the other relevant literature. They should discuss instances in which their findings differed from those of other researchers, suggest possible reasons why, and offer interpretations of their findings. For example, if the study found that the more time children spent outside daily was associated with improved test scores, what can you take from this in terms of policy and practice? What still remains to be learned? Importantly, the Conclusion section should also discuss the scope and limitations of the study. All studies have limitations, and you want to read critically to see that there are no sweeping generalizations or contributions attributed to the findings that are not attributable to the data or analysis (Dunifon, 2005). You need to be sure the claims that are made are realistic. For instance, unless a study contains a randomized experiment, it is difficult to determine cause and effect. Even without knowing the specific statistical formulas and so on, you can appraise whether or not a sweeping generalization was made or if cause was attributed when this was not the goal of a study. In addition, you can review when there may be other variables at play that may not have been identified as limitations (e.g., did reduced screen time really cause children's test scores to rise, or was it something else, such as lesson plans or variables in the social or family environment that the researchers were not able to observe?). You will want to ask these specific questions in your appraisal of the limitations, discussion, and conclusions:

- How does the researcher overcome the limitations of the method? Are there significant or minor limitations? How will these limitations affect your ability to use the data to answer your research question?
- Did the researcher find a correlation (relationship) or a cause?
- Are there alternative interpretations of the findings?
- How generalizable are the findings? Can the findings be applied to other populations or situations? What contribution does the study make to the advancement of knowledge, theory, or practice?

HOW DO I WRITE A RESEARCH CRITIQUE?

There are many ways you can compose a written research critique. Instruction will likely be provided in an assignment, and you may be asked to compose the work in a formal essay with an abstract, introduction, body, and conclusions format with headings and general features of an essay or academic paper. Writing a research critique typically follows the seven steps listed in box 5.2.

These broad guidelines and steps for writing a research critique address only some of the concerns and questions you will explore in your reading and review of research articles. More specific research appraisal guidelines and checklists are provided in chapters 6 and 7 and in the appendices. Developing a clearer picture of the purpose and practical steps of reading and appraising what you read will build your research literacy and expand how you can communicate about research for practice.

Box 5.2: Steps for Writing a Research Critique

1. Start by identifying the article's title, authors, date of publication, and name of the journal or other publication in which it appeared. In your introduction, briefly describe the purpose and nature of the study and, if applicable, its theoretical framework (see table 5.1). If the paper was not published in a peer-reviewed journal, consider the credibility of the publication in which it appeared and the credentials (and possible biases) of the researchers.

2. Organize the body of the written critique according to the structure of the research paper you are reviewing. Consider the ideas in this chapter, the guidelines in table 5.2, as well as specific guidelines in chapters 6 and 7 for suggestions about questions to ask in your critique of various elements of different research articles. Start with a brief description and analysis of the strengths and weaknesses of the research design and methodology and then critically review the presentation and interpretation of the findings and the researchers' conclusions. If the research topic is time sensitive, consider whether the data used in the study was sufficiently current.

3. Use headings to structure your critique. In each section, provide enough descriptive information so that your review will be clear to a reader who may not have read the study.

4. Aim to develop an objective, balanced, and well-supported critique. Polit and Beck (2017) advise that you maintain a balance by pointing out the strengths and weaknesses of the research paper and justifying your criticism by giving examples of the study's weaknesses and strengths.

5. Conclude your critique by briefly summarizing the strengths and weaknesses of the study and by assessing the study's contribution to the advancement of knowledge, theory, or practice. Consider suggesting research directions and methodological considerations for future researchers.

6. Use past or present tense consistently whenever you refer to completed research. Check if your professor or institution has a preference for which tense they'd like you to use in the text.

7. Use a standard citation style, such as APA (2010), *MLA Handbook* (Modern Language Association, 2016), or Chicago/Turabian (University of Chicago, 2010), to format references in your critique, and be sure to cite page numbers for all quoted passages.

REVIEW AND REFLECT

The purpose of this brief overview of the appraisal process was to broadly introduce how to conduct a critical reading and review of a research paper. While there are some guidelines and specific steps for this process, there are many different approaches to research and distinct methodologies and methods. There is no one tool that will be appropriate or sufficient as a guide for your reviews. In chapters 6 and 7, you will proceed to refine your critical review skills and to better understand different approaches: qualitative, quantitative, and mixed methods. Taken together, these chapters are a useful resource for navigating through the volumes of research you are able to examine.

Although it may be difficult at times to sift through longer or more complex research papers, there are many benefits of staying up-to-date and critically appraising what is known on a topic. By reading original research, you can draw your own conclusions as to the relevance of research findings to your everyday practice. Research can be used to update both the design of community programs and existing resource materials. As a result, with a critical eye, you can act as an informed practitioner and can begin to integrate major findings from research into your work in health and community practice.

6 | HOW DO I UNDERSTAND AND INTERPRET QUALITATIVE RESEARCH PAPERS?

"Not everything that can be counted counts, and not everything that counts can be counted."

—William Bruce Cameron

LEARNING OBJECTIVES

This chapter focuses on knowledge that will enable you to identify qualitative research, qualitative research questions, and the ways data are gathered, interpreted, and analyzed. You will move from this general understanding to interpreting the findings in a qualitative study and to being able to appraise the research. It will enable you to start thinking about how you could use these research methods to improve your own professional practice. After reading this chapter and completing the practical learning activities in appendix B, you will be able to do the following:

- Describe the key characteristics of qualitative research.
- Describe the methodologies used in qualitative research.
- Explain the meaning of the results of a qualitative study.
- Judge the results to determine trustworthiness.
- Explain how research results help you to provide care or service for your clients in health and community practice.

CHAPTER OUTLINE

- Key Characteristics of Qualitative Research
- Methodologies Used in Qualitative Research
- Examples of Research Studies Using Various Qualitative Approaches
- How Do I Know if Qualitative Results Are Trustworthy?
  - Rigour (Trustworthiness) in Qualitative Research
- Example of a Completed Qualitative Research Report Appraisal
- When Do I Use Qualitative Research in Practice?
- Review and Reflect

KEY CHARACTERISTICS OF QUALITATIVE RESEARCH

Some of the background that relates to qualitative and quantitative research and how these relate to different worldviews (paradigms) were introduced earlier in chapter 2. The concepts of qualitative (non-numerical) and quantitative (numerical) data were also introduced earlier in chapter 4. To read qualitative research papers, you need a sound understanding of the concepts specific to this type of research to make full sense of the report.

Qualitative research recognizes that there are social and cultural influences on how people experience the world. As well, qualitative research assists us with our understanding of the world (Patton, 2015, p. 2). This form of inquiry is mostly concerned with the process of the research rather than the outcomes, and is interested in understanding how people make sense of their lives, experiences, or phenomena. Qualitative research is defined as "the investigation of phenomena, typically in an in-depth and holistic fashion, through the collection of rich narrative materials using a flexible research design" (Polit & Beck, 2017, p. 741). Health and community practice is informed and influenced by humanistic philosophy, which stresses the socially constructed nature of reality, the intimate relationship that exists between people and the situational constraints that shape practice. Consequently, qualitative research for health and community practice is expected to pay attention to both the holistic belief system and the value of the contextual circumstances in interpreting research participant experiences. Therefore, qualitative research becomes particularly appropriate for health and community practice, especially when the intent is to obtain an account of personal in-depth perspectives or experiences. For example, if the phenomenon of interest is a better understanding of those living in poverty in a particular community, several different research approaches could be used. A survey could be used to collect data on the rate of poverty within this community; however, it may not easily capture the particular social, cultural, or political factors that may be contributing to their poverty. As a result, another way to gain a deeper understanding and appreciation of those who are living in poverty within this community is to enter the environment in which these people live. The researcher could go into the field and interview people regarding their experiences and perspectives as well as observe their life experiences. Then the researcher becomes part of the setting in which the data are collected. However, it is important to acknowledge that there is subjective bias. Later in this chapter, *rigour*, as it relates to the researcher being part of the study, will be discussed. The data collected will be words of text (qualitative) rather than numerical data (quantitative) to describe how poverty is experienced and interpreted by this particular community. Using a qualitative approach for understanding the complexities of living with the human phenomena of "poverty" allows for participants to describe what they experience, which is not easily quantifiable. In this example, qualitative research can draw from the theoretical perspectives, such as critical social theory, that illuminate the social construction of knowledge, while acknowledging the importance of the context where the phenomena is experienced. Some other examples of the theoretical perspectives used in qualitative research include critical theory, post-colonial theory, feminist theory, and symbolic interactionism. This is not an all-encompassing list; for more theoretical perspectives and in-depth explanations, we suggest you consult other research textbooks. In qualitative research, this inductive approach for knowledge development is based upon "generating new concepts, explanations, results, and/or theories from the specific data of a qualitative study" (Patton, 2015, p. 67).

In summary, the characteristics of qualitative research include the following:

- People's varying realities
- The importance of participants' perspectives
- Acknowledgement that the researcher is part of the study
- The importance of the context
- The collection of narrative data that are used to describe, analyze, and interpret participants' perspectives
- An ongoing analysis of the data being collected

METHODOLOGIES USED IN QUALITATIVE RESEARCH

Within qualitative research, there are different approaches (methodologies), which were briefly discussed in chapter 3. For instance, in the humanistic exploration of a client's experiences of homelessness services, a client may be asked directly about his or her experiences of receiving different support services. A researcher undertaking a study on this topic may adopt one of these approaches:

- Follow a particular group over a prolonged period of time—in the past this would have involved living among that population (this is known as *ethnography*).
- Explore what clients understand about the services and build a theory as the research progresses (*grounded theory*).
- Explore the lived experience of receiving housing support services (*phenomenology*).

There are a variety of approaches used in qualitative research.

It is important to understand that with these approaches, there is variability in the philosophical or disciplinary origins and the specific types of research questions that will be explored. In terms of sampling, it is often purposive and data collection is undertaken through various forms, such as interpersonal interviews, fieldwork observation, and reviewing documents (Patton, 2015). Data analysis is an inductive approach, with ongoing comparisons looking for themes and patterns in the data, and in the case of grounded theory, the emergence of a theory. It is important to emphasize that the chosen approach must align with certain requirements of that method. In addition, you will read about other types of qualitative research—for example, case studies, narrative analysis (Clandinin, 2007), descriptive qualitative studies, and interpretive description (Thorne, 2016).

EXAMPLES OF RESEARCH STUDIES USING VARIOUS QUALITATIVE APPROACHES

Table 6.1 describes the three qualitative approaches, types of questions asked, philosophical or disciplinary origin, sample, how data are collected, focus on the findings, and how the data are analyzed.

To further understand what studies in these qualitative approaches in table 6.1 look like, you may find the following examples helpful (see boxes 6.1, 6.2, and 6.3).

Table 6.1: Qualitative Approaches

Common Approaches	Origins	Question	Sample	Data Collected	Findings	Data Analyzed
Ethnography	Anthropology	What is the culture of the group of people?	Purposive, non-probability	Fieldwork: observations, field notes, document reviews, interviews	Describing the culture as experienced by the group (culture)	Describing the interpretation of the meaning of the groups in their cultural context
Grounded theory	Social sciences	What is the theory that explains what is being observed?	Purposive, theoretical sampling	Interviews, participant observation, document reviews	Describing the emerging theory	Comparative analysis—ongoing (iterative), looking at actions and processes
Phenomenology—descriptive or hermeneutical approaches	Philosophy	What is the meaning of the lived experience?	Purposive	Multiple interviews	Description of the experience by the participant; interpretation of the experience by the researcher; themes	Dependent upon whether a "descriptive" or "hermeneutical" approach was used

Box 6.1: Qualitative Approach—Ethnography Example

Qualitative Approach: Ethnography.

Question: To explore how clients in residential care experience surveillance technology (ST) in order to assess how ST might influence autonomy.

Sample: Purposeful sampling; two long-term residential care facilities for people with intellectual disabilities (42 clients) and interviews with six people (family and staff); and a nursing home for people with dementia (43 clients) and interviews with eight people (family and staff).

Data Collected: Participant observation combined with conversations with clients and interviews with family and staff.

Findings: A pattern of two themes:

- Theme One: "Coping with new spaces," which entailed clients wandering around, getting lost, being triggered, and retreating to new spaces.
- Theme Two: "Resisting the surveillance technology measure" because clients feel stigmatized, missed the company, and do not like being "watched."

Conclusions: ST used in residential care requires critical evaluation and reflection of how each individual ST measure is experienced by clients; therefore, the clients are not left alone, but the aim is staff support and to give meaning to all ST-related activities of people with intellectual disabilities and dementia.

Source: Based upon "The Experiences of People with Dementia and Intellectual Disabilities with Surveillance Technologies in Residential Care," by A.R. Niemeijer, M.F.I.A. Depla, B. Frederiks & C. Hertogh, 2015, *Nursing Ethics, 22*(3), pp. 307–320. Copyright 2015 by Niemeijer et al.

Box 6.2: Qualitative Approach—Grounded Theory Methodology Example

Qualitative Approach: Grounded Theory.

Question: To broadly explore maternal perceptions of mother–infant communications among low-income, primiparous mothers in the Southeastern United States using the grounded theory methodology (GTM), and to subsequently frame findings in the context of potential impacts on compliance with infant feeding recommendations.

Sample: A total of 15 participants; purposeful sampling.

Data Collected: In-depth telephone interviews.

Analysis: The researchers used Charmaz's (2006) grounded theory approach, with coded transcripts analyzed using constant comparison emergent techniques (reflexivity log, memoing, open-ended questions during the interviews, and theoretical sampling). This process allowed themes and the central concept to emerge and lead to impending saturation.

Findings: The central concept or phenomenon resulted in a theoretical model of "Mother–Infant Communication Dynamic" (Waller, Bower, Spence & Kavanagh, 2015, p. 749) and three main themes interconnected with this phenomenon:

- Theme One: Perceived infant development and communication capabilities. The following example narrative supports this theme: "When they're newborns ... they can't do much body language or ... so new at it, you don't understand what cry in which ... as they get older, I guess you get used to it and into a routine of ... things" (Waller et al., 2015, p. 755).

- Theme Two: Maternal focus influencing maternal response. The following example narrative supports this theme: "[I]'m out of the state where I was worried about SIDS ... and they say it peaks at 3–4 months, and so once I got that out I felt comfortable ... because you worry about every little thing as a new mom, and I'm sure any mom really. But now it's keeping him happy, and of course health, but um helping him meet his milestones; like he can sit up now by himself with you know little pillows around him, and ... just kind of fostering a learning environment now, now that he's old enough and wants to interact more with things" (Waller et al., 2015, p. 755).

- Theme Three: Resulting feeding practices. The following example narrative supports this theme: "When she was first born she woke up probably every hour and a half ... consistently. She never slept through the night, not even close, until about six months and then she'd wake up 2 times a nights so it just took her a long time to slept through the night; nothing, no cereal, not solid foods, none of that helped" (Waller et al., 2015, p. 755). This theme included four underlying interconnected, supporting concepts: hectic guessing game, starting to understand, better interaction, and speaking the same language.

Conclusions: This study found that during the first year of life a communication pattern results in the maternal perception of mother and infant speaking the same language, which may result from inaccurate maternal interpretations of infant behaviours and cues and may lead to inappropriate infant feeding practices. The researchers suggest that further research is needed to test this theoretical model in other ways, for example, direct observation of mother–infant communication to understand maternal interpretation of infant cues that could potentially use these concepts to attenuate excess rapid infant weight gain.

Source: "Using Grounded Theory Methodology to Conceptualize the Mother–Infant Communication Dynamic: Potential Application to Compliance with Infant Feeding Recommendations," by J. Waller, K.M. Bower, M. Spence & K.F. Kavanagh, 2015, *Maternal and Child Nutrition, 11,* pp. 749–760. Copyright 2015 by Waller et al.

Box 6.3: Qualitative Approach—Phenomenology (Using Descriptive Method)

Qualitative Approach: Phenomenology (using descriptive method).

Question: To explore immigrant Chinese women's experiences in accessing maternity care, the utilization of maternity health services, and the obstacles they perceived in Canada.

Sample: 15 participants, purposeful sampling.

Data Collected: In-depth unstructured interviews.

Analysis: As this was a "descriptive phenomenology study" (Lee et al., 2014, p. 1), the researchers used a Colaizzi's (1978) phenomenological method to analyze the data.

Findings: Six themes emerged:

1. Preference for linguistically and culturally competent health care providers, with obstetricians over midwives. The following example narrative supports this finding: "I am worried about the process of delivery. I feel safe if someone can explain to me what's going on using the language I understand" (Lee et al., 2014, p. 4).

2. Strategies to deal with the inconvenience of the Canadian health care system. The following example narrative supports this finding: "I phoned the OB's [obstetrician's] clinic which I preferred. After confirming they had openings for new patients, I then requested my family physician to refer me to the OB" (Lee et al., 2014, p. 4).

3. Multiple resources to obtain pregnancy information. The following example narrative supports this finding: "I often check the Chinese websites if I need to know something" (Lee et al., 2014, p. 5).

4. Merits of the Canadian health care system. The following example narrative supports this finding: "Here in Canada it is better because it's one-to-one when your doctor examines you at prenatal visits. Back home there were often some other women waiting inside the examining room and overheard the conversation between you and your doctor" (Lee et al., 2014, p. 5).

5. Need for culturally sensitive care; this is related to cultural practices. For example, following birth, "in Chinese tradition, a woman should not touch anything cold after birth" (Lee et al., 2014, p. 5).

6. Emergence of alternative supports and the use of private services. The following example narrative supports this finding: "My own mother couldn't come due to a visa issue and my husband didn't know how to cook, so we hired a Yue-Sao. She stayed three hours every morning for a month to cook Zuo Yue Zi meals for me. She was a nurse back

home, so she is professional and knowledgeable. She is my consultant for postnatal practices" (Lee et al., 2014, p. 6).

Conclusions: This study found two unique experiences of "preference for linguistically and culturally competent health care providers, with obstetricians over midwives, and the emergence of alternative supports and the use of private services" (Lee et al., 2014, p. 9). The researchers suggest that further research is needed with women of other cultural backgrounds to develop a complete understanding of immigrant women's health services needs during the time period of pregnancy, childbirth, and the postpartum period.

Source: "A Descriptive Phenomenology Study of Newcomers' Experience of Maternity Care Services: Chinese Women's Perspectives," by T.-Y. Lee et al., 2014, *BMC Health Services Research, 14,* pp. 1–9. Copyright 2014 by T.-Y. Lee et al.

HOW DO I KNOW IF QUALITATIVE RESULTS ARE TRUSTWORTHY?

Reading qualitative research papers and appraising the value for your practice requires many of the steps of the general research critique process, as discussed in chapter 5. In addition, critical appraisal of qualitative research papers involves some particular questions and examinations that relate to the specific paradigm and methodologies as well as the kinds of research questions that are explored in a qualitative research project. While reading and appraisal guides could be established for each and every kind of research study in qualitative and quantitative methodologies attending to the technical differences in each study, the value of a basic foundational approach to reading and appraising qualitative papers is presented here for those seeking basic foundational skills. Qualitative and quantitative research begins from unique philosophic assumptions so these approaches to research do have distinct tasks for reading, understanding, and appraising the quality of the study, as noted in table 6.1. The 13 main questions to be considered in your reading (appraisal) of qualitative research papers are listed in table 6.2.

Table 6.2: Questions to Ask When Reading Qualitative Research Papers

1. Citation	What is the name of the paper? The complete citation?
2. Purpose and study rationale	Did the authors provide a clear statement of the aims of the research?
3. Fit and specific rationale	Is a qualitative methodology appropriate?
4. Design	Was the research design appropriate to address the aims of the research?
5. Participants	Was the recruitment strategy appropriate to the aims of the research?
6. Researcher (or researchers)	Has the relationship between researcher and participants been adequately considered?
7. Ethics	Have ethical issues been taken into consideration?
8. Context	Where did the study take place?
9. Data	What was the sequence of the study? Were the data collected in a way that addressed the research issue?
10. Analysis	Was the analysis of the data sufficiently rigorous?
11. Findings and results	Was there a clear statement of findings?
12. Conclusions	What did the authors assert about how the results and study process contribute to the conclusions?
13. Implications and application	How valuable is the research?

Source: Adapted from "Understanding and Critiquing Qualitative Research Papers," by P. Lee, 2006, *Nursing Times, 102*(29), pp. 30—32, and from *Reading and Understanding Research* (3rd ed.), L.F. Locke, S.J. Silverman & W.W. Spirduso, 2010, London, United Kingdom: Sage.

Rigour (Trustworthiness) in Qualitative Research

Ensuring adequate "rigor in qualitative research is important in demonstrating to the respective publics who read qualitative research that it is a respectable approach to science" (Streubert & Carpenter, 2011, p. 48). There is also no one process for ensuring rigour or trustworthiness appropriate for all qualitative studies, but generally the goal of rigour is to accurately represent study participants' experiences (Rolfe, 2006).

The following criteria for evaluating qualitative research were outlined originally by Lincoln and Guba (1985):

1. Credibility entails activities that ensure that trustworthy findings will be produced, which enables readers to have more confidence in them. Examples of *credibility* include (a) prolonged engagement with the topic being studied and (b) member checking data, whereby the findings are returned to the participants for validation of accuracy (Streubert & Carpenter, 2011, p. 48). *Triangulation processes* are another way of enhancing credibility of the conclusions in qualitative studies.

    There are four kinds of analytical triangulation: (a) *triangulation of qualitative sources*, which looks for consistency across interviews; (b) *mixed qualitative-quantitative methods triangulation*, which looks for consistency of results produced by different data collection methods; (c) *analyst triangulation*, which calls for other analysts to review the results; and (d) *theory/perspective triangulation*, which uses multiple theories or perspectives to make sense of the data (Patton, 2015, p. 661). Consult with other research textbooks for more in-depth descriptions of the specifics of these triangulation processes (refer to the Further Resources and Links at the end of this text).
2. Dependability is established once the researchers have provided the credibility of the findings (Streubert & Carpenter, 2011, p. 49).
3. Confirmability encompasses the documentation of an *audit trail*, which is an ongoing record of the process that was followed and the decisions that have been made during the research study (Streubert & Carpenter, 2011, p. 48).
4. Transferability (also known as *fittingness*) is the ability of the findings to have meaning and be applicable in other similar situations (Streubert & Carpenter, 2011, p. 48).

The main goal of qualitative research is to provide a rich and contextualized understanding of the human experience. In order to capture real experiences and to reflect an authentic image of those experiences, careful appraisal of the value of the research contribution is important when deciding on the application of those findings to practice. The appraisal of rigour in qualitative research can be challenging, as students often equate such an appraisal with quantitative research (Locke et al., 2010).

The fittingness, auditability, credibility, trustworthiness, and saturation (FACTS) strategy supports a quick and comprehensive appraisal of the rigour and trustworthiness in qualitative research papers (El Hussein, Jakubec & Osuji, 2015). FACTS is summarized in table 6.3 and discussed in more detail below.

Table 6.3: FACTS for Appraising Rigour in Qualitative Research Papers

F	Fittingness
A	Auditability
C	Credibility
T	Trustworthiness
S	Saturation

Source: Based upon "Assessing the FACTS: A Mnemonic for Teaching and Learning the Rapid Assessment of Rigor in Qualitative Research Studies," M. El Hussein, S. L. Jakubec & J. Osuji, 2015, *The Qualitative Report, 20*(8), pp. 1182–1184.

In the FACTS mnemonic, *F* for *fittingness* (also termed *transferability*) is the ability of the researcher to demonstrate that the findings have meaning to others in similar situations (Beck, 1993). Transferability is dependent on the degree of similarity between two contexts (Koch, 1994). Sandelowski (1986) further elaborated, "A study meets the criterion of fittingness when its findings can [fit] into contexts outside the study situation and when its audience views its findings as meaningful and applicable in terms of their own experiences" (p. 32). The *A* in FACTS is for *auditability*, which is about maintaining a comprehensive record of all methodological decisions, such as a record of the sources of data, sampling, decisions, and analytical procedures and their implementation. This is sometimes referred to as *confirmability*. Guba and Lincoln (1989) termed this record an "audit trail" (p. 243). The *C* in FACTS stands for *credibility*, which relates to "the extent that the research methods inspire confidence that the results and interpretations are truthful" (Polit & Beck, 2017, p. 161). Guba and Lincoln (1989) suggest that a study is credible when it presents such a vivid and faithful description that people who had that experience would immediately recognize it as their own. The *T* in FACTS is for *trustworthiness*, which is a concept in qualitative research that encompasses all of the above-mentioned steps (El Hussein et al., 2015, p. 1183). Trustworthiness reflects the quality of a research report and ascertains that the necessary steps have been taken and thoroughly described to ensure that the study procedures meet high standards and that results can be trusted. Finally, the *S* in the mnemonic is for *saturation*. Data saturation in qualitative research occurs when the researcher no longer hears or sees new information. This could also be referred to as *informational redundancy*. Dey (2007) used the analogy of a soaked sponge that cannot hold or contain more water to explain saturation; once achieved, "adding ... further ... data makes no difference" (p. 185).

EXAMPLE OF A COMPLETED QUALITATIVE RESEARCH REPORT APPRAISAL

Based upon the questions presented in table 6.2 (Questions to Ask When Reading Qualitative Research Papers) and the research methodology from box 6.2 (Qualitative Approach—Grounded Theory Methodology Example), box 6.4 illustrates possible responses to the questions for a review of the paper.

Box 6.4: Critical Review of a Qualitative Research Paper—A Grounded Theory of Infant Feeding

1. *Citation: What is the name of the report? What is the complete citation?*
    It is important to first look for the completed elements in the citation of the qualitative study. This should include authors, date of publication, title of the study, and the journal, volume, and page numbers. Subsequently, the other questions to ask regarding these elements are, Does the title of the research align with the journal chosen for publication? For example, in box 6.2, the "title" of the study, which focuses on infant feeding, aligns with the content that one might expect in this journal. The complete citation can be listed in a standard referencing format. The following reference citation is in the APA publication style (American Psychological Association, 2010):

    > Waller, J., Bower, K.M., Spence, M., & Kavanagh, K.F. (2015). Using grounded theory methodology to conceptualize the mother–infant communication dynamic: Potential application to compliance with infant feeding recommendations. *Maternal and Child Nutrition, 11,* 749–760. http://dx.doi.org/10.1111/mcn.12056

2. *Purpose and study rationale: Do the authors provide a clear statement regarding the aims of the research?*
    Somewhere, generally early in the research paper, the authors should describe what the study is about, and include some of the background as to why the study is valuable and important. The problem or origins for the research should be discussed in a way that clearly points to the purpose and rationale for the research (versus just embarking on a program or policy to address the problem being experienced).
    Waller et al. (2015) provide a detailed "Introduction" section in which they describe the purpose (i.e., the reason why they conducted

their study, followed by how they conducted the study). Waller et al. describe how rapid weight gain in early infancy has been linked to the risk of obesity and being overweight in later life, which can be associated with other chronic conditions such as type 2 diabetes. The authors explain that conducting this study would be helpful for better understanding what types of feeding recommendations could be instituted. This background provides a clearly stated research question that relates to the significance of the study and how the knowledge gained from this study would be used in the future.

3. *Fit and specific rationale: Is a qualitative methodology appropriate?*
Based upon the background information, you must then decide whether a qualitative approach appears congruent with what the researchers desire to study.

   In this study, the researchers state that the process of infant feeding practices is complex, and that there is a need to understand the factors that influence how these decisions occur, which is unknown (Waller et al., 2015).

4. *Design: Was the research design appropriate to address the aims of the research?*
As the researchers were interested in the generation of a theory (Waller et al., 2015), the grounded theory qualitative approach was appropriate.

5. *Participants: Was the recruitment strategy appropriate to the aims of the research?*
An important element for the grounded theory approach is theoretical sampling. Waller et al. (2015) clearly followed Charmaz's (2006) model, which is a well-known practice guide used for constructing grounded theory.

6. *Researcher(s): Has the relationship between researcher and participants been adequately considered?*
In qualitative research, anonymity is not possible as the participants are known to the researcher; therefore, their identities must be safeguarded. The researchers in this study responded to this by ensuring that ethical guidelines were adhered to throughout the study (Waller et al., 2015). (Refer to question 7 for more details of what was done to specifically address this.)

7. *Ethics: Have ethical issues been taken into consideration?*
    The researchers state clearly that the study had received ethical approval from their university Institutional Review Board. In addition, they describe in sufficient detail the process followed for recruitment of the participants. The recruitment process was voluntary, and all potential participants for the study were fully informed regarding what was required of them for the telephone interview (Waller et al., 2015).

8. *Context: Where did the study take place? What happened, where, and when? What was the sequence of the study? How vivid are the representations of the context?*
    In qualitative research papers, it is essential that vivid descriptions and portrayals of affect with illustrative examples that show the investigator's purpose are presented. How will you make an appraisal of the expression of this context? Firstly, you will read the report carefully and determine if you will resonate with what is expressed—or not.
    The researchers conducted telephone interviews, so the context in this particular study would be the place where the participant was situated, which was not explicitly discussed. The researchers, however, in the "Strengths and Limitations" section of their report, acknowledged that the telephone interviews prevented direct observation of the mother–infant interactions (Waller et al., 2015, p. 758).

9. *Data: Were the data collected in a way that addressed the research issue?*
    You should find the presentation of actual data in a qualitative research paper. The data are usually embedded in the description of what was done in the study and how the conclusions were drawn. Data are often presented in a brief format—for instance, in selected quotations, short textual examples, photos, and so on.
    This study clearly provides a descriptive diagram of the theoretical model of "mother–infant communication dynamic" (Waller et al., 2015, p. 749), tables of the participant characteristics of sample (p. 753), tables with quotations from the participants of the supporting concepts (p. 755), and the three themes and the central phenomenon (p. 755). Sufficient detail is provided to get a sense of the meaning of the data collected.

10. *Analysis: Is the analysis of the data sufficiently rigorous?*
    It can often be difficult to know if the data analysis was rigorous, particularly if you are unfamiliar with the specific analysis method.

In addition, rigour in qualitative research differs from the processes in quantitative research. As the researchers specifically describe that a grounded theory approach was used (Waller et al., 2015), you could anticipate that an appropriate process for analyzing the data was followed. As stated under Question 5, the researchers used Charmaz's (2006) theoretical model, which is an appropriate analytic strategy to use for this study. If you are unsure whether a particular analysis strategy is appropriate for a study, refer to a more comprehensive research textbook or consult a researcher familiar with qualitative research methods.

Rigour in qualitative research is often described by discussing the credibility, dependability, confirmability, and transferability of the inquiry (Guba & Lincoln, 1989). The researchers address in detail areas of rigour in the "Strengths and Limitations" section (Waller et al., 2015). Specifically, they discuss the consistency; inter-coder reliability; purposeful sampling strategy to achieve a homogenous sample, providing strength to the findings for the particular sample, which was comprised of low-income, first-time, urban mothers living in one specific area of the country; and the rigorous and systematic analysis used for the grounded theory approach as outlined by Charmaz (2006) to provide dependability (Waller et al., 2015). (Please review the previous section in this chapter for discussions of rigour in qualitative research.)

11. *Findings and results: Is there a clear statement of findings?*
The researchers provide numerous clearly described examples of the findings in both tables and narrative form, along with what their results mean (Waller et al., 2015).

12. *Conclusions: What do the authors assert about how the results and study process contribute to the conclusions?*
Waller et al. (2015) were able to take the findings of the "mother–infant communication dynamic" (p. 749) and apply this to practice.

13. *Implications and application: How valuable is the research?*
In the "Conclusions" section of the report, the authors clearly describe the next steps for research through building on the theoretical model by using direct observation of the mother–infant communication, which may increase the understanding of maternal interpretation of infant cues that may influence infant weight gain.

WHEN DO I USE QUALITATIVE RESEARCH IN PRACTICE?

As previously alluded to in this chapter, qualitative research will be used in practice when you are interested in understanding how an individual experiences a particular phenomenon, rather than how it is measured (see table 6.4 for examples of questions you might explore in a qualitative approach).

Table 6.4: Examples of Qualitative Research Questions You Might Consider Answering in Your Practice

Qualitative Approach	Example of Research Question
Ethnography	How does international development work with clients impact those with HIV/AIDS who have been abandoned by their families in Ghana?
Grounded theory	How can the process of deciding to migrate to another country for work be understood?
Phenomenology	What is the lived experience of families who are homeless and are living in a shelter?

REVIEW AND REFLECT

Careful examination of qualitative research gives interprofessional practitioners a better understanding of how a group of people or individuals view, understand, and bring meaning to a particular experience. It can, therefore, enable individual practitioners to expand their skills and contribute to evidence-informed practice. Moreover, interprofessional practitioners who have the knowledge to appropriately and effectively evaluate and apply qualitative research will broaden their ability to improve the quality of care provided in health and community practice. In addition, these skills will help them better communicate with others in the social and humanity fields.

7 | HOW DO I UNDERSTAND AND INTERPRET QUANTITATIVE RESEARCH PAPERS?

"Quantitative research should begin with an idea (usually articulated as a hypothesis) which then, through measurement, generates data and, by deduction, allows a conclusion to be drawn."

—Trisha Greenhalgh

LEARNING OBJECTIVES

This chapter focuses on knowledge that will enable you to identify quantitative research when you encounter it in your own reading and help you to evaluate and understand the methodologies used. It will also enable you to start thinking about how you could use these research methods to improve your own professional practice. After reading this chapter and completing the practical learning activities in appendix B, you will be able to do the following:

- Describe the key characteristics of quantitative research.
- Describe methods used in quantitative research.
- Explain the meaning of the results of a quantitative study (e.g., what are p-values, what is a confidence interval).
- Explain how these results will help you to provide care or service for your clients in health and community practice.

CHAPTER OUTLINE

- Key Characteristics of Quantitative Research
  - Hypotheses
  - Cause and Effect
- What Methods Do Quantitative Research Studies Use?
  - Quantitative Research Methodology
- What Are the Results of a Quantitative Study? How Are Quantitative Research Studies Analyzed?
  - Statistics
- How Do I Appraise a Quantitative Research Paper?
- Review and Reflect

As introduced in chapter 3, there are a number of reasons researchers undertake a study using deductive reasoning and the quantitative paradigm. Determining whether an intervention does what it claims to do is a key component to quantitative methods in health and community practice. The debate around the use of supplements or cold remedies is an everyday example of the type of question for quantitative examination. Regardless of the purpose, these studies need your careful appraisal. If a client uses supplements and feels better, the client may think that the remedy is the cure. You might then ask the question, "If the client took the remedy and got better, does it matter whether the remedy worked or not?" Indeed, this is a reasonable response, but what if the remedy were toxic or expensive? Many modern medicines and treatments are expensive and many have a host of side effects, and sometimes the medication or treatment has no significant effect. The question then becomes, "Why take or encourage treatments that are costly and have no benefits, or that may actually be worse than doing nothing at all?" Avoiding unnecessary expense and side effects are two reasons why it is important to undertake experimental or other quantitative studies. Such questions require experimental approaches to answering them and demonstrate why these approaches are highly encouraged in evidence-informed practice.

Experiments and quasi-experiments are types of research that are performed to test cause and effect. The cause (or independent variable) is manipulated, or introduced, by the researcher under carefully controlled conditions, and the effect (or dependent variable) is then measured. Experiments and quasi-experiments are widely used to test the usefulness of educational programs in increasing understanding, clinical interventions in improving clinical outcomes, screening to identify disease, and the changing of methods of care delivery and services to improve the care or treatment experience and satisfaction. The characteristics, key terms, and considerations for appraisal of quantitative research will be discussed briefly in this chapter.

KEY CHARACTERISTICS OF QUANTITATIVE RESEARCH

Quantitative research methodologies are used to answer questions that have a numerical, quantifiable element to them, or that set out to prove an association between two variables that cannot be described as having a cause and effect. Essentially, quantitative methodologies fall into one of two broad classifications: those that are interventional (or experimental) and those that are observational.

Interventional studies seek to manipulate an exposure (the independent variable) in order to measure what effect it has on an outcome (the dependent variable). For example, a study could be performed analyzing physical literacy education for seniors (the independent variable or exposure) to improve their balance and decrease falls (the dependent variable or outcome). Observational studies, on the other hand, seek to explore the associations between a naturally occurring independent variable (exposure) and a dependent variable (outcome; Gordis, 2008). This is because it is not always possible to be certain regarding causation, often because there may be several potential causes contributing to an effect. Some of these causes will be known and some will not. It is necessary, therefore, to be more cautious when assigning a cause. The terms *association*, or sometimes *correlation* (although this also has a strict research meaning, as you will see in the glossary), are used instead. For example, there may be an association found between violent television viewing during preschool years (the independent variable or exposure) and later childhood aggressive behaviour (the dependent variable or outcome), even though childhood aggressive behaviour could also be associated with other environmental and social factors.

Researchers *operationalize* or provide rules and definitions to establish change or measurement. A definition gives meaning to a concept by specifying the activities necessary to measure it (e.g., if a study is measuring student success based on caffeine consumption, the terms "student," "success," and "caffeine consumption" must all be defined). It should be clear in the quantitative research papers you are reading exactly what the variables are in the study.

The *independent variable* (IV) is generally defined as the variable that influences the dependent variable. It is any variable that defines different groups of participants who are measured via the dependent variable. It can also be a variable that describes the qualities of the participants. The *dependent variable* (DV) is the variable that is hypothesized to change in response to the IV. It is the variable that is hypothesized to be *influenced by* the IV. Refer to the chapter learning activity in appendix B for more practice.

Hypotheses

When conducting an experiment, it is good practice to start with a hypothesis. A *hypothesis* is quite literally an idea that is less than or below (*hypo*) a proposition or idea (a *thesis*). That is, it is an idea that has yet to be tested or proven using the scientific method. A hypothesis, then, is a statement that explores the relationship between at least one dependent and one independent variable that is empirically tested. An example of a general hypothesis could be "women's education level affects childbearing." A more specific hypothesis could be "as a woman's education level increases, the number of children she will have decreases." Box 7.1 shows the important characteristics of a hypothesis.

Box 7.1: Characteristics of a Hypothesis

- Suggest the relationship among the variables.
- Identify the nature of the relationship.
- Point to the research design to be used.
- Indicate the population to be studied.

Hypotheses are often arrived at as the result of either experience or clinical observation, and as an outcome of qualitative research or other observational research. They remain theoretical until proven otherwise, and even once "proven," they remain open to further study. In an experimental study, the researcher manipulates one or more independent variables to see what happens to the dependent variable. In its simplest form, this means manipulating one independent variable in one group of participants and measuring the change in a dependent variable (often called a pre-post-test or before-and-after study).

Cause and Effect

A *cause* is simply something that has an effect. In quantitative research terminology, it is common for a number of terms to be used for cause and effect, but essentially quantitative research is interested in causes (independent variables or exposures) and effects (dependent variables or outcomes). As a result, we can describe the same event in one of three ways:

1. Increased falls (effect) may result from poor physical literacy (cause).
2. Increased falls (dependent variable) may result from poor physical literacy (independent variable).
3. Increased falls (outcome) may result from poor physical literacy (exposure).

We can assess the relationship between the dependent and independent variables through measurement. This might be through temperature, weight, speed, and cortisol levels, as examples.

Confounding occurs when there are alternative explanations for an outcome in a study that are not taken into account. Confounding variables are always independently associated with both the exposure and the outcome being measured. For example, an increased risk of pancreatic cancer (the dependent variable studied) is associated both with smoking (the independent variable studied) and with coffee drinking (an independent variable not studied), and smokers tend to drink more coffee than non-smokers.

These measurements and deeper understanding of the nature and realities of cause and effect allow health and community practitioners to intervene in a meaningful way in the lives of individuals and communities. For example, having an understanding of the cause of falls supports community health practitioners in meaningful health promotion choices regarding physical literacy or other interventions (such as interventions to a client's environment), or both, depending on what are concluded to be the cause and effect of falls.

WHAT METHODS DO QUANTITATIVE RESEARCH STUDIES USE?

In chapter 6, you learned that the researcher is seen as a tool of data collection in qualitative research, which provides a depth and richness to the process (Patton, 2015). This personal engagement to the collection of data is necessary to understand the human interactions that form the basis of qualitative research. You also learned that because of the interactive nature of the data-collecting methods in qualitative research, it is hard to eradicate bias in qualitative research (Patton, 2015).

The collection of data within the quantitative methodologies requires researchers to be one step removed from the process so that they remain objective and their approach to the process is consistent. This detachment ensures that the quality of the data collected is high and that there is less room for *bias* (the introduction of systematic errors) to creep into the data-collection process. Quantitative methodologies are concerned with numbers, with understanding associations between variables, and with demonstrating cause and effect. Gathering such data requires researchers to engage in much thought, not only about what information they want to collect, but also about how they might collect it and how they might ensure the quality of the process. The key feature of all quantitative study methods is the consistency and accuracy of the data-collection process. Methods in quantitative studies are always concerned with the consistency (or *reliability*) and accuracy (or *validity*) of the data collection to ensure that the data collected are suitable for generalizations. *Validity* refers to accuracy and how well a measure assesses what it claims to measure. For instance, if *a survey used in a research study is supposed to measure quality of life, how is that concept defined? Is it measurable?* Extensive discussions of reliability and validity are available in several texts (see, for example, Creswell, 2014).

The specific and well-defined nature of outcome measures means that the results of quantitative research are often capable of being generalized (i.e., applied with a fair degree of certainty outside of the research setting). Unlike qualitative research, which moves from the specific observation toward the generation of more general hypotheses, the purpose of quantitative research is to move from general observations to the generation of more specific outcomes.

Generalizability is an important feature of quantitative research because it allows the researcher and user of the research to have a fair degree of certainty that the research findings apply to subjects that have the same, or broadly similar, characteristics as the participants involved in the study. Think of it this way: as a health and community practitioner, it is important that you feel the services and care you offer to your clients and communities will be effective and safe. For example, it is important for practitioners to know that the techniques for workplace stress management taught or the diabetic teaching advice given will be effective. This knowledge is generated by research that has been carried out to demonstrate this efficacy.

If research has involved people who are broadly similar to the clients in your service, you can have some certainty that the information you apply from the research will be relevant to your clients and their unique circumstances. The same research will not apply to people with different needs or from a different set of circumstances. For example, the research may have taken place in only 100 people with diabetes or workplace stress, but it applies to those whose situations are broadly similar to the people who took part in the research.

Quantitative Research Methodology

There are a number of questions that quantitative research methods can be used to answer and, like qualitative methods, there are a number of issues that are not the focus of a quantitative study. The key questions that may be explored by quantitative methodologies are outlined in table 7.1. The approaches to a research study and data collection methods correspond to the questions that are asked. It should be recognized that there are considerable overlaps in methods, and often multiple data-collection approaches are used in a study, a practice known as *triangulation*.

The different research methodologies and associated methods of data gathering each have different advantages and disadvantages. Given that each methodology and method of data collection has its weaknesses, it makes some sense for researchers to employ a variety of approaches within their research in order to minimize the impact of these failings. Therefore, for example, a brief questionnaire might lead to a focus group, which might lead to one-on-one interviews. Using such techniques not only allows the data collected to be enriched but also compensates for any weaknesses or biases in the methods employed for the study.

Table 7.1: How Different Quantitative Methodologies Can Answer Research Questions

Questions	Methodology
If x is done, what will happen?	Experiment or quasi-experiment
If x is done, how often will y happen?	
If a person is exposed to x, will they develop outcome (disease) y?	Randomized controlled trial (RCT)
Does exposure to x cause outcome y?	Cohort studies
What exposure x might have caused this individual to have outcome y?	Case-control studies
In this group of people, how many have been exposed to x or have outcome y? What is the prevalence of x or y in this group?	Ecological studies
The data show that when x increases in the population so too does y—might they be associated?	Cross-sectional studies
When exposure x increases and outcome y increases, is there potential that the two are associated in some way?	Experimental and quasi-experimental research

Experiments for health and community practice are not the same as experiments that take place in a laboratory. Rather, these experiments involve the researcher (or experimenter) examining the relationship between two variables. For example, does increased education about diet alter food choices in an isolated community for people with diabetes? These experiments are carried out prospectively (i.e., data are collected in real time and do not rely on memory or old notes) in an attempt to prove cause and effect. The reason that any experiment is conducted is because there is genuine uncertainty about which treatment is best for the participants. This is called the uncertainty principle (described in chapter 1), and "best" in this context might be taken to mean cheapest, safest, most effective, or easiest to use.

Observational studies, such as case-control and cross-sectional studies (which are those that involve no intervention on the part of the researcher), often lead to the generation of ideas that can be tested using experimental study designs. Sometimes it is difficult to know which of two variables in an observational study caused the other to happen (if, indeed, they are at all related). A good example of this may be breastfeeding women with mastitis who receive antibiotics; do they get better because of the antibiotics, or because of their immune systems? Another example is the administration of educational interventions and a student's learning outcome. In this case, are learning outcomes improved because of the educational intervention, or other variables such as student intelligence, socioeconomic background, and personality traits impacting the student's ability to learn and hence the outcome? These studies will measure variables before intervention (e.g., student learning before educational intervention) and again after intervention (e.g., student learning after educational intervention).

Case-Control Studies

Case-control studies compare people with a specific disease or outcome of interest (cases) to people from the same population without that disease or outcome (control). *Case series*, on the other hand, are studies that report observations on a series of individuals, usually all receiving the same intervention, with no control group. Case-control studies seek associations between the outcome and prior exposure to particular risk factors (e.g., one group may have been exposed to a particular substance that the other was not). They are usually concerned with causes of a disease and are generally retrospective.

The sample for a case-control study is taken by selecting people who have an outcome of interest, such as lung cancer, and pairing them with appropriately matched individuals who do not have the outcome of interest. Cases need to be well defined. It is not enough, for instance, to define your sample as people with hypertension (high blood pressure); it is better to state what is meant by high blood pressure (e.g., greater than 150/85 mmHg on three consecutive occasions). It is also important to define where the cases are from (their source) because this provides information about how representative the sample is of all people with the outcome of interest. Controls must also be chosen with care. If the aim of the study is to compare like with like, then the controls need to be very similar in all respects, other than not having the disease, to the case population.

Data collection for case-control studies are usually undertaken by studying clinical or other documentary records, by interviewing (the cases and controls or their relatives), and by taking, or using existing, biological samples. One of the major problems with case-control studies, and a good reason why they are generally used to generate hypotheses that are later tested in prospective studies, is that they often rely on participant recall, which is not always vivid or accurate—a phenomena known as *recall bias*. Recall bias can prove to be a major obstacle in the execution of any study. It arises in a number of ways, all of which are systematic. For example, people who had a bad experience in childbirth will be more likely to remember it in a negative fashion, as compared to people who had a positive childbirth experience, who will conversely remember the experience as being good. Mothers of children with birth defects are more likely to recall the use of alcohol and smoking during pregnancy than mothers whose children are born healthy, as another example.

Cross-Sectional Studies

A *cross-sectional study* is essentially a snapshot phenomenon at a point in time. This kind of study cannot be used to demonstrate the incidence or prevalence of an exposure or an outcome in a given group of individuals, unlike the prospective methods discussed earlier. *Incidence* describes the risk of contracting a disease or condition, whereas *prevalence* indicates how widespread the condition is within a given population. Often researchers use the two terms interchangeably, but they are not synonymous.

Cross-sectional studies are useful for planning the delivery of a service and for estimating future needs. They are very common in health and community practice research and are quick, inexpensive, and easy to conduct. Cross-sectional studies allow researchers to generate hypotheses that can be tested using other quantitative methods such as random control trials and cohort studies. Surveys are a form of cross-sectional study that may be used to discover any number of things, including demographic data, the presence or absence of disease, and people's opinions, views, and values. It is standard practice for universities to collect data on students' opinions of their courses and instruction; this is a simple cross-sectional study usually undertaken for quality monitoring (audit) purposes. Since data on exposures and outcomes are collected simultaneously, cross-sectional studies are not good at demonstrating a sequence of events. For example, a cross-sectional study of mental illness and unemployment would be difficult to interpret since it is likely that mental illness is both a cause and effect of unemployment. Due to this challenge, cross-sectional studies are considered to be one of the weaker study designs.

The sample for a cross-sectional study is usually drawn from a population in which the exposures or outcomes of interest are known to be fairly prevalent. Data for cross-sectional studies are often drawn from pre-existing evidence, such as blood test results, data held on institutional databases, or information held by local authorities. Such data may be supplemented during the course of a study by taking biological samples, by using questionnaires, or by conducting structured interviews.

Quasi-Experimental Studies

Quasi-experimental studies are concerned with comparing measurements and are usually applied to the observation and measurement of changes that occur naturally (sometimes called natural experiments). Herttua, Mäkelä, Martikainen, and Sirén (2008) reported that a dramatic decrease in the price of alcohol in Finland in 2007 (independent variable) did not lead to an increase in violence (dependent variable). It may seem odd to think that this is an example of an experiment because there is no manipulation of any variable by the researcher. However, when you consider that it might be impossible, or unethical, to undertake certain experiments on a large group of subjects (e.g., to make large volumes of alcohol available to a large group of people to measure its effects on their behaviour), then the benefits of the natural experiment become more apparent.

Quasi-experiments rely solely on the measurement of unmanipulated independent and dependent variables. As there is no control over the environment in which the study takes place, there is a real danger that the outcomes of such studies are affected by factors that are unknown to the researchers. Consequently, the results of such research studies must be treated with great caution. When working with such data, there is a real need to be certain that there is some plausibility to the associations being made. Data collection in experimental and quasi-experimental studies depends on the exact question under investigation. The data collected can include information about the independent variable, such as demographic data (e.g., age, gender, and ethnicity), which may be collected from pre-existing sources including databases or individuals themselves, and data on a phenomenon (e.g., a sports injury or natural disaster), which may be found in chart documents, collected from news sources, or gathered especially for the study by interview or questionnaire. Outcome (dependent variable) data may also be collected from existing records or may be gathered especially for the study using data collection methods such as interviews, questionnaires, and physical examinations.

The sample (the individuals to be studied) chosen for an experimental or quasi-experimental study depends on the question posed in the hypothesis, as well as on the design and methods of the study. For example, consider a study on acupuncture used for pain relief. First, it is important to define what constitutes pain and what part of the body is affected before identifying a study sample. In this case, let us say the study is an intervention (acupuncture) specific for the treatment of neck pain following a motor vehicle accident (MVA). There is a need to sample people from the population that exist with this condition (post-MVA neck pain), but there may also be a need to be more precise in defining the sample so that the effects of acupuncture specific to this group are what is actually measured and described. The research sample may then be more specifically focused on people experiencing a *first incident* of neck injury from MVA, and those who have no previous neck pain. The outcome of the study would, therefore, apply only to people with the specified injury and not to other people seeking acupuncture to treat pain from other causes or injuries.

Once these criteria are met and a large population is identified, individuals for the study may then be chosen from that population—this is called the study sample. When the selection process gives everyone in the larger population the same chance of participating in the study (so long as they meet the other criteria), this is called *probability sampling*, and when the sample size is big enough (often calculated using statistical formulae), a sample that is representative of the larger population has been produced. In a natural experiment, the sample for the study includes the people who have experienced the phenomenon under investigation but are exposed to the experimental or controlled conditions by nature or factors not in the control of the researchers. Natural experiments are most useful when it would otherwise be unethical to run a true experiment or when there has been a clearly defined exposure involving a well-defined sub-population (and the absence of exposure in a similar sub-population).

Randomized Controlled Trials

In health and community practice, *randomized controlled trials* (RCTs) are specifically used to determine cause and effect and are often used to demonstrate the effectiveness of a therapeutic intervention. RCTs use a number of methods for collecting the study data. These methods include clinical and non-clinical measurements (e.g., blood cholesterol levels, wound healing rates, participant satisfaction, and quality-of-life data). Problems with undertaking RCTs in the practice setting include time, ensuring that the trial protocol and procedures are followed correctly, and keeping accurate records of all study interventions.

In RCTs, two or more interventions are compared by being randomly allocated to participants. RCTs may include a control intervention or no intervention and if possible should be single or double blinded. Blinding involves preventing those involved in a trial from knowing to which comparison group (i.e., experimental or control), a particular participant belongs. With blinding, the risk of bias is minimized. In double-blind experiments, participants, caregivers, outcome assessors, and certain researchers can all be blinded (although this is not always feasible). An example of this type of RCT may be the study of whether patient-controlled analgesia improves patient satisfaction with the first week of recovery post-hip-replacement surgery when compared to standard pain medication administered by injection every four hours.

Cohort Studies

Unlike the experimental study designs, *cohort studies* do not involve an intervention on the part of the researcher—they are purely observational. Cohort studies are observational studies of selected groups measuring selected variables over time. Outcomes are compared to examine subjects who were either exposed or not exposed to a particular intervention. Cohort studies are said to be able to determine the causality of disease (i.e., they are able to link exposure to a certain independent variable with the disease being researched). A retrospective cohort study identifies subjects from past records and follows them to the present, while a prospective cohort study assembles participants and follows them into the future. Prospective studies are considered stronger than retrospective studies as there may be less of a concern with recall bias, which leads to questions about whether the study demonstrates what it claims.

As with RCTs, there remains the need for a comparison group in a cohort study so that it is possible to compare exposure in one group to non-exposure in the other, and thus determine the extent to which the outcome of interest is caused by the exposure (demonstrating causality). There are many issues relating to how and who is selected to be in the comparison group. There is a need to keep the two groups as similar as possible in order for the only difference between the two groups to be the exposure to a variable that is then analyzed in the outcome. In studies such as the Nurses' Health Study (NHS), this is achieved by studying a large homogeneous (largely similar) group of nurses of similar ages and, when an outcome of interest arises, comparing the data on exposures between those who have the outcome (or disease) of interest and those who do not. In more specific cohort studies, a comparison group would be drawn from people who are largely similar to the group under investigation, except that they are not exposed to the potential cause.

The most frequently used data collection method in cohort studies is self-completion questionnaires. The use of self-completion questionnaires is driven by the fact that these studies are large and take place over a long period of time. As a result, individual visits, or data collection by study staff, can be very expensive and time consuming. One famous, large, and longstanding cohort study is the NHS, which has examined women's health in three large cohorts over many years (see box 7.2).

Box 7.2: The Nurses' Health Study Cohort Research Project

The world's largest, longest running *study* of women's *health* is a cohort study research project known as the NHS. The first Nurses' Health Study (NHS I) started in 1973 and its scope and cohort size were further expanded in 1989. In 1976, the study enrolled married registered nurses, aged 30 to 55, who lived in 11 US states. Of the 170,000 nurses initially approached, approximately 122,000 nurses responded. Every two years, all members of the cohort received a follow-up questionnaire regarding diseases and health-related topics, including smoking, hormone use, and menopausal status. Every four years since 1980, the cohort also received questions relating to their dietary habits, and since 1990, questions about quality of life have been added. Response rates to the questionnaires were high, at about 90 percent. A second study (NHS II) was started in 1989 with younger participants (aged 25–72 years) to study emerging areas of interest such as contraception use, diet, and lifestyle data. The cohort for this study was somewhat smaller at around 117,000 participants. In 2008, NHS III was initiated, again to a younger generation of nurses.

Major findings of the Nurses' Health Studies include the following:

- Birth control pills do not increase non-smoking women's risk of heart disease.
- Women who take oral contraceptives for more than five years have less than half the risk of ovarian cancer than women who have never used birth control pills.
- Women who take estrogen after menopause decrease their risk of heart disease, but raise their risk of developing breast cancer.
- Increased dietary calcium intake among post-menopausal women is not protective against fractures of the hip and wrist, although a positive

relationship has been observed between protein intake and risk of fractures.

- A diet rich in red meat raises the risk of colon cancer.
- Women who drink moderate amounts of alcohol (one to three drinks per week) cut their risk of heart attack in half, but increase their risk of breast cancer by one-third.
- Limiting fat intake and eating more high fibre foods does not reduce a woman's risk of breast cancer.
- Women who have taken multivitamin supplements that contain folic acid have a 75 percent reduced risk of colon cancer.

Source: Nurses' Health Study, by Brigham and Women's Hospital, Harvard Medical School & Harvard T.H. Chan School of Public Health, 2016, Boston, MA: Harvard University.

Ecological Studies

Ecological studies are a kind of epidemiological study in which the unit of analysis is a population or community (defined in various ways) rather than an individual. For instance, an ecological study may look at the association between smoking and lung cancer deaths in different countries. Disease rates and exposures are measured in each of a series of populations and their relationships are examined. Often the information about disease and exposure is abstracted from published statistics and therefore these studies do not require expensive or time-consuming data collection.

WHAT ARE THE RESULTS OF A QUANTITATIVE STUDY? HOW ARE QUANTITATIVE RESEARCH STUDIES ANALYZED?

Quantitative data are generated through the variety of methods described previously and can be measured and analyzed in a number of ways. Statistics are the primary approach to analysis of quantitative data (Polit & Beck, 2017). Given the variety and number of statistical tests available, it is beyond the scope of this textbook to present all of these here; rather, key approaches to analysis are discussed in general in this chapter. Specific measures are sought through more distinct techniques, and are often achieved through computer-assisted statistical analysis software.

Statistics

Many people believe that without graduate-level statistics courses they will be unable to interpret results in a research paper. Your skills in critical appraisal should not be seen as simply statistical know-how; "this misconception often leads to an overestimation of the level of statistical knowledge required for critical appraisal" (Ajetunmobi, 2001, p. 1). What is needed to understand statistics is only your logical thinking ability to comprehend the concepts (Polit & Beck, 2017). Nonetheless, a little statistical knowledge can help you to better understand and use quantitative research.

Statistics are all around us. In fact, it would be difficult in our world today to go through a full week without using statistics. Imagine watching a hockey game where no one kept score and game statistics. Beyond our recreational activities, without statistics we could not plan our budgets, determine differences between outcomes from one intervention or another, evaluate performance of equipment or tools, or perform a host of other practice-relevant issues. We need statistics, but do not let these numbers and tools trouble you—they are just that: tools. A basic statistics textbook can help you understand any quantitative analysis at a fundamental level. Sophisticated understanding is rarely important for your reading or use of a quantitative paper. Still, be patient with yourself, seek clarity, and do not let the statistics trip you up!

Descriptive Statistics

Different data types can be presented in different ways using descriptive statistics. *Descriptive statistics* do exactly what they say—they describe patterns of data within a data set. Descriptive statistics are used to give the reader some idea of the make-up of a study, the numbers of people involved, and their spread of age, gender, and ethnicity, for example. The exact data to be presented depends on the nature and purpose of the study undertaken and will, therefore, vary. Descriptive statistics are concerned with the presentation of summaries of data generated during a study. Examples of the ways in which descriptive statistics are presented include basic calculations, graphs, charts, and tables. Descriptive statistics can be used in your reading and for your current practice. You probably already know more about these statistics than you think. For instance, you are likely familiar with the terms *mode*, *mean*, and *median*.

The concept and uses of mode answer the question, "Which score appears most often in our data set?" The *mode* is the most frequently occurring number in a set of observations. When people speak of a "middle" score they often think of what is known as the *mean*, or the *average* of a set of scores. The mean is calculated by adding all of the values in a data set together and then dividing by the number of values. For example, all the ages of the people involved in the study divided by the number of people involved in the study would give us the mean age.

Mean and median can be a little confusing, because both of them measure a type of "average" score, we call them measures of *central tendency*, or measures of the centre of the scores in a given data set (Gerstman, 2015). *Median*, specifically, is a measure of the *middle score* of a group of scores. For example if a data set has 21 scores, then the 11th score in the ordered set is the median score.

The *variance* of a sample measures how the scores are spread around the mean. Large variance means the scores are widely spread around the mean. Variance is a measure that poses a slight problem. When you are using variance, you are dealing with squares of numbers. This makes it a little hard to relate the variance to the original data, so how can you "undo" the squaring that took place earlier? The way most statisticians choose to do this is by taking the square root of the variance—known as the *standard deviation*. The standard deviation enables the researcher and reader to get a feel for where most of the variables within a data set lie. In a normal distribution, 66 percent of all the data will lie within one standard deviation of the mean, while 95 percent of observations will lie within two standard deviations (Gerstman, 2015). The reporting of the mean and the standard deviation of a given data set allows the researcher and readers of the research to get a good feel for where most of the values within the data set lie.

By looking at many different measures, you can discover more about a given data set. One such measure is known as the *range*. In order to get a better idea of how a given data point relates to other data, it is important to get an idea of how the data are spread out. The *range* is the distance between the highest and lowest data points in a set.

Inferential Statistics

Descriptive statistics are used to reduce a data set of numbers into a few uncomplicated values that are represented either as numbers or in graphs. In this sense, descriptive statistics are like a book summary—they get across the basic idea without the detail. The purpose of *inferential statistics* within the research process is to demonstrate that the findings of the research extend beyond the sample within which the research was carried out. What this means is that despite the fact that the findings are not 100 percent certain, we can place a fair degree of confidence in the statistical findings of any quantitative research.

The findings of inferential statistics are usually expressed in terms of probability. The probability to which they refer is the likelihood of the findings of the study being found by chance. In other words, probability shows us how much confidence we can have that the findings of the study did not occur purely by chance. Probabilities are expressed as *risk, p-values,* and *confidence intervals* (Gerstman, 2015). In the reality of everyday practice, even a small knowledge of these basic inferential statistical concepts will be sufficient to appraise most quantitative papers.

Risk

What is the measure of *risk*? Simply put, the risk of something happening is its chance of occurring. It tells us about the chance of something happening, but it is not a guarantee that it will happen. It may be confusing, comparing something like a risk of "7 out of 35" with a risk of "3 out of 10" (3 out of 10 is a bigger risk in this example). With the numerous ways that risk is talked about this can be very confusing for your clients in practice—and perhaps for you too! All the more reason to develop a strong basic literacy in statistics; this will enable you to support others in interpreting and acting on the risk statistics as presented in any given study. To add to your literacy and ability to communicate risk to your clients, it is important to remember that different ways of describing the same risk can profoundly affect how that risk is perceived. The actual risk itself is often referred to as the *absolute risk*. The higher the absolute risk is, the more likely it is that the something will happen—although it still is not guaranteed to take place. Comparing two risks, a researcher will come up with a *relative risk* to find out how much more likely one is compared to the other (Gerstman, 2015).

These risks can be expressed as odds ratios or risks ratios. An *odds ratio* (OR) is a measure of association between an exposure and an outcome. The OR represents the odds that an outcome will occur, given a particular exposure, compared to the odds of the outcome occurring in the absence of that exposure (Szumilas, 2010). While the OR expresses the odds of an event occurring in two groups (those with the exposure and those without), the *risk ratio* (RR), or weighed mean difference, expresses the ratio of the risk of an event in the two groups. For ease of understanding, people talking about risk often use percentages (although many people are confused by the presentation of data in percentages as much as numbers or other scores). A percentage simply tells us the number of times something happens out of every 100 chances, and allows risks to be compared more easily. In our earlier case of 7 out of 35 versus 3 out of 10, these can be converted into 20 percent compared to 30 percent.

The following are all statements of the relative risk of developing cancer: "People who use indoor tanning beds are 20% more likely to develop malignant melanoma" and "one alcoholic drink per day increases breast cancer risk by 5%." These statements tell us how much more, or less, likely a disease is in one group, compared to another. However, they do not tell us anything about the overall likelihood—or the absolute risk—of any of these things happening at all. The size of the initial absolute risk is what is really important here. If the initial risk is very small, even a huge increase may not make much absolute difference, but for a risk that is quite large already, smaller increases can still have a big impact (Gerstman, 2015).

Let us go back to real-life research examples to see how much difference this can make. A study published in 2012 demonstrated that having several computed tomography scans as a child could make that child three times more likely to develop leukemia or brain cancer as an adult (Pearce et al., 2012). This sounds alarming (and scarier still, another way of saying three times as likely is a 200 percent increased chance). However, digging a little deeper into the research demonstrates that, because the chances of developing these cancers are so small (0.4 per 10,000 children aged 0–9 develop brain tumours and 0.6 per 10,000 children aged 0–9 develop leukemia), the increased risk would actually mean one additional case of brain cancer and one of leukemia for every 10,000 children given the scans.

To make informed decisions, you, and your clients, need to know what the risks *actually* are, and how they compare to each other. As a health and community practitioner, it is often your responsibility to assist your clients in understanding what these risks really mean and subsequently the actions that ought to be taken.

The results from any particular study will vary just by chance, and you must be cautious in reading results and relaying the findings to clients. Studies differ in terms of the people who are included (the sample), and the ways in which people react to the intervention or exposure. Even when everything possible is held constant, there will still be some random variations. As a result, there are statistical tools to help the researchers assess whether differences between new and old treatments in any particular study are real and important, or just manifestations of chance variability. Confidence intervals and *p*-values help do this.

p-Values

The *p*-value stands for the probability that a result could have occurred by chance if, in reality, the null hypothesis was true. If a result is statistically significant, it will be indicated by a *p*-value. In the case of this value, a scale is assigned to the rating of probability that something will occur, ranging from zero to one. The *null hypothesis* is the topic of study (the exposure or intervention; for instance, acupuncture) that has no impact on outcome (e.g., post-motor vehicle accident neck pain). A *p*-value of less than 0.05 would mean the likelihood of the results being due to chance is less than 1 in 20, so the effect of the intervention or exposure would be considered statistically significant (Gerstman, 2015). In this way, a statistically significant result means that the exposure or intervention (such as acupuncture) is believed to create the effect and not chance.

Confidence Intervals

The *confidence interval* is the plus-or-minus figure that describes the margin of effect for the results. This corresponds to hypothesis testing with *p*-values, with a conventional cut-off for *p* of less than 0.05. For example, in a literacy study examining the number of correctly completed disability benefits applications, it was determined the mean is 77 percent with a confidence level of 95 percent, and the confidence interval is 70 percent to 84 percent. Therefore, if the data are sampled 1,000 times, in 95 percent of those samples, the average of those successfully completing the disability benefits application will fall between 70 and 84 percent.

If the confidence interval is narrow, capturing only a small range of effect sizes, you can be quite confident that any effects far from this range have been ruled out by the study. This situation usually arises when the size of the study is quite large and, therefore, the estimate of the true effect is quite precise. Another way of saying this is to note that the study has reasonable power to detect an effect. However, if the confidence interval is quite wide, capturing a diverse range of effect sizes, it can be inferred that the study was probably quite small. In this case, any estimates of effect size will be quite imprecise. Such a study is considered to have a low power or strength and ultimately provides less information from which to base decisions. In assessing the importance of significant results, it is the size of the *effect*, not just the size of the significance, that matters.

The *confidence level* tells you how sure you can be about a given result. It is expressed as a percentage and represents how often the true percentage of the population who would pick an answer lies within the confidence interval. A 95 percent confidence level means you can be 95 percent certain; a 99 percent confidence level means you can be 99 percent certain. Most researchers use the 95 percent confidence level (Gerstman, 2015). When you put the confidence level and the confidence interval together, you can say that you are 95 percent sure that the true percentage of the population falls within a certain range. The wider the confidence interval you are willing to accept, the more certain you can be that the whole population's answers would be within that range.

There are three factors that determine the size of the confidence interval for a given confidence level: sample size, percentage, and population size. The larger a *sample size*, the more certain you can be that scores truly reflect the studied population. This indicates that, for a given confidence level, the larger the sample size, the smaller the confidence interval. Accuracy also depends on the *percentage* of the sample that picks a particular answer (Gerstman, 2015). If 99 percent of a sample said, "Yes," and 1 percent said, "No," the chances of error are remote, irrespective of sample size. However, if the percentages are 21 percent and 79 percent, then the chances of error are much greater.

As a researcher increases the confidence level, for example, from 95 to 99, the confidence interval gets larger. In other words, in order to be more confident that the interval actually contains the population mean, a researcher has to increase the size of the interval, that is, to be less precise. The trade-off between level of confidence and the precision of our interval then happens by increasing the sample size. *Population size* is only likely to be an issue impacting the confidence interval with a relatively small and known group of people (e.g., the members of an association). The confidence interval calculations, however, assume there is a genuine random sample of the relevant population. If the sample is not truly random, you cannot rely on the intervals (Gerstman, 2015). This is why a reader of research will appraise these key aspects of a quantitative study.

HOW DO I APPRAISE A QUANTITATIVE RESEARCH PAPER?

Reading quantitative research papers will expand your ability to critically appraise research articles. Many different tools can guide your appraisal, including those discussed in chapter 5 and those available in the additional resources and links provided at the end of the text. You can begin the process of appraisal by asking some basic questions. The 13 general steps are listed in table 7.2.

REVIEW AND REFLECT

Quantitative research studies generally analyze questions about cause and effect. These studies demonstrate quantifiable measurements that all have a numerical element. This chapter described the main quantitative methodologies used in health and community practice research. The choice of study design is influenced by a number of issues that include the nature of the question asked, whether the study is attempting to show cause and effect (experimental designs and cohort studies), and whether the study is looking for potential associations (case-control studies) or merely measuring the prevalence of a phenomenon (cross-sectional studies). We have seen that samples used in various studies have to be carefully chosen and described in order to maintain the validity of a study and that various data-collection methods are used in order to generate the findings for a given research methodology.

Table 7.2: Questions to Ask When Reading Quantitative Research Papers

1. Citation	What is the study report? The complete citation?
2. Purpose and study rationale	Did the authors provide a clear statement of the aims of the research?
3. Fit and specific rationale	Is a quantitative methodology appropriate?
4. Design	Was the research design appropriate to address the aims of the research?
5. Participants	Was the recruitment strategy appropriate to the aims of the research? Are the sampling issues relevant to the methodology adequately addressed? Does the sampling strengthen or weaken the quality of the results?
6. Researcher (or researchers)	Has the relationship between researcher and participants been adequately considered?
7. Ethics	Have ethical issues been taken into consideration?
8. Context	Where did the study take place?
9. Data	What was the sequence of the study? What constituted data (e.g., test scores, questionnaire responses, etc.) and were data collected to address validity and reliability concerns?
10. Analysis	What form of data analysis was used, and what specific question was it designed to answer? What statistical operations and computer programs were employed?
11. Results	What are identified as the primary results (products of findings produced by the data analysis)?
12. Conclusions	What did the authors assert about how the results and study process contribute to the conclusions?
13. Implications and application	How valuable is the research? Consider generalizability and any limitations.

Source: Adapted from *Reading and Understanding Research* (3rd ed.), L.F. Locke, S.J. Silverman & W.W. Spirduso, 2010, London, United Kingdom: Sage.

It is important to bear in mind, however, that if practice is to be established or changed on the basis of some quantitative research, it is imperative that the research stand up to critique. Critical appraisal is necessary before applying findings in practice. Refer to the chapter 7 learning activities in appendix B for more practice.

When reading quantitative research, you should be aware that quantitative data collection requires a specific and predetermined protocol. The sample size should be large—the larger the better. The quality and consistency of data collection and recording outside research are variable and should be evaluated to determine the strength of the findings. Data analysis is statistical and should describe trends, compare groups, and relate variables. The analysis should also compare results with past research.

Decisions for applying new research to practice and for making decisions or changes in practice are always based on a number of factors, and the quality of the evidence is just one part of that choice. Review the evidence-informed decision-making model from chapter 1, and refer to chapters 8 and 9 to consider more of the application of quantitative research in your practice.

8 | HOW DO I KNOW WHAT IS BEST EVIDENCE FOR PRACTICE?

"Be skeptical. But when you get proof, accept proof."

—Michael Specter

LEARNING OBJECTIVES

This chapter focuses on the skills necessary for appreciating and understanding evidence for application in practice. After reading this chapter and completing the practical learning activities in appendix B, you will be able to do the following:

- Describe what is considered the best evidence according to the evidence pyramid or hierarchy of evidence.
- Explain how policies, protocols, and clinical guidelines contribute to evidence for practice.
- Evaluate what may be considered best evidence.
- Describe how a knowledge translation model can assist with the uptake of evidence.

CHAPTER OUTLINE

- Skepticism and Critical Appraisal for Practice Decisions
  - What Is Considered Best Evidence?
  - Evidence Pyramid or Hierarchy of Evidence
  - Knowledge Syntheses and Systematic Reviews
- What Is Best Practice?
  - Benefits of Practice Guidelines
  - Potential Limitations of Clinical Practice Guidelines
- How Do Policies, Protocols, and Guidelines Contribute to Evidence-Informed Practice?
  - Adapting Guidelines for Practice
- Review and Reflect

As a student or interprofessional practitioner, it is important to acknowledge that one study is rarely a reason to make immediate changes to your practice. As discussed in chapter 7, trends or associations do not necessarily indicate a causal relationship or warrant changes in your practice. Often new research does not provide statistically significant findings or generalizable applications to practice. In addition, findings may be refuted or, as contexts and circumstances change, the findings that were once applicable may now not be applicable to a new context or population. Practice decisions and advice, particularly decisions that have implications (e.g., for clients, populations, or society), should not be based solely on one study. Instead, it is important to evaluate the overall results available and track patterns over time in order to come up with well-supported guidelines for decisions in your practice. Once you finish your studies, you will often be asked for advice as a professional based on what is known—health and community practitioners are often asked for such advice both in professional and personal situations. If you are still in doubt after referring to summaries of the best evidence (e.g., if there are conflicting summaries), then further scrutiny and analysis are needed. In the end, the best advice is always to be skeptical and to consider the broader evidence-informed practice considerations.

SKEPTICISM AND CRITICAL APPRAISAL FOR PRACTICE DECISIONS

It is smart to look at every research paper with a healthy dose of skepticism and to be careful when explaining the findings or potential generalizability to your practice area. Be mindful that many studies in health and community practice are exploratory, and may only suggest correlations or associations, not causality. The findings may certainly be of value, and contribute to knowledge on a subject or problem, but as readers and users of research for practice, be cautious about accepting claims made or considering application of findings or recommendations. There is a big difference between a report that *proves* A causes B, versus one that simply *links* A and B. For example, children who consume carbonated drinks high in sugar may have a greater incidence of attention deficit hyperactivity disorder (ADHD), but this could be due to chance alone. Another example is the infamous, and now discredited, 1998 *Lancet* study by Wakefield et al. that claimed that the MMR vaccine was linked to autism. The news reports from this research paper frightened some parents into not vaccinating their children. As a result, there was an increase in the cases of measles in many communities, causing serious health problems for many children and deep tension and dilemmas for many parents. Other factors, such as the expiry date of the vaccination, the typical age of diagnosis for autism, and the age when children are vaccinated with the MMR vaccine, make causation difficult to prove. These confounding variables (as explained in chapter 7) must be considered when reading research papers and considering practice decisions. Detecting bias in research papers is also important. Was the research sponsored by a drug company, or could other factors contribute to bias?

All research (potentially) provides evidence, but there are no perfect studies. As a result, systematic processes need to be in place to appraise and evaluate the efficacy of a research paper. For example, critical appraisal involves a standardized review of research to judge the quality, trustworthiness, and relevance (Burls, 2009). To provide the best possible practice, the strongest evidence is needed to support health and community practice decisions and action. Critical appraisal (as introduced earlier in chapter 5) of articles, books, reports, and other sources will help evaluate any biases or methodological shortcomings that may be present and help build that larger, compiled story to determine if changes in practice are warranted.

For example, a systematic review "uses a rigorous process (to minimize bias) for identifying, appraising and synthesizing studies to answer a specific clinical question and draw conclusions about the data gathered" (Melnyk & Fineout-Overholt, 2015, p. 611). Based upon the conclusions, practitioners will decide how they might apply changes to their practice context. Critical appraisal is a central tenet of the systematic review and is used in evidence-informed practice to assist in making decisions. In reading the research, whether rigorous systematic reviews, RCTs, economic evaluations, or other research, remember to consider the following questions first: What is the study's relevance for your practice (or within the context of knowledge synthesis for your area of health or community practice)? Remember also that if your goal is to understand beliefs and meanings in the group with whom you are working, then qualitative studies can be important. As a result, other methods used to evaluate qualitative studies will need to be explored in more detail in other research textbooks.

Acquiring critical appraisal skills is essential for all studies, including systematic reviews, particularly in an era of information overload. There are several appraisal guides or tools to assist you in this important step (see the tools and websites referenced in the Further Resources and Links section at the end of this textbook). As noted in chapters 5, 6, and 7, questions for your critical appraisal of research can take a number of forms, asking very specific questions for both qualitative and quantitative research papers (see table 6.2 for a listing of questions to ask when reading qualitative research papers and table 7.2 for questions relating to quantitative research). Research literacy means being aware of the value of research for practice, with an understanding that you must read critically with an eye for the relevance to your practices and to common limitations for the applicability of research to your practice.

There are general credibility and agenda (bias) questions you can ask on an initial review for a research paper. It is doubtful that any study of health or community relevance would be totally without some kind of bias, either in the study design or in the author's pre-existing beliefs. In particular, consider these elements:

- Question bias: Examine the question being addressed and consider what kind of research gets funded.
- Publication bias: Research that shows no effect tends not to get published.
- Conflict of interest, author affiliation, and sources of funding: Does the researcher have a vested interest in the outcome?
- Documentation and assumptions: Are all stated facts referenced?
- Peer review: Is the article peer-reviewed? Does it matter?
- Authority: Does the researcher have the knowledge to work in this area?
- Significance of a single study: Science is an incremental process; one study rarely changes everything.

In general, a beginning appraisal will focus on basic questions (for some first-level appraisal questions, see box 8.1).

Box 8.1: Five First-Level Critical Appraisal Questions

1. Has the topic been researched before? Was the literature reviewed? How were data collected before? Is there a need for this study in your field (e.g., to explore the research questions with a larger or different population)? Are there areas of study that need further exploration? Does the study add anything new to the body of literature?
2. Was the research conducted with strong, clear methods? Was the research conducted in ways that minimize bias (e.g., control groups for interventions, blinding, or randomization in a quantitative study, and member checks and reflexivity in qualitative analysis)?
3. Does the study question or population relate to your health and community practice area?
4. What does the study tell you? Are the results applicable to other contexts?
5. What will the results mean for your health and community practice problem or questions when decisions must be made?

These questions will assist you in reading research papers for basic practice relevance and applicability. For more in-depth critical appraisal questions for the qualitative and quantitative research papers you will read, please use the respective critical appraisal guidelines in appendix B.

What Is Considered Best Evidence?

Appraisal of research or evidence has become complex and daunting. Is best evidence revealed by the number of research studies that show the same things? What about the quality of the research done? People must draw conclusions about the quality of evidence and strength of recommendations before taking up any recommendations in practice. Systematic and explicit approaches to appraisal and acquiring the available evidence can help protect against errors, resolve disagreements, and assist in sorting through the volumes of, often conflicting, evidence. Researchers must effectively communicate information and fulfill actual needs for practice (perhaps to change practitioner behaviour or direct where resources are best spent); however, wide variation in approaches to the appraisal of the evidence derived from research exists. Regardless of the appraisal approach, one begins with a healthy dose of skepticism, and then there are also some common views of what lowers quality of evidence. Learning about these dimensions is helpful as a critical reader and user of research for practice. Here are some key quality control considerations:

- Methodological limitations
- Inconsistency of results
- Indirectness of evidence
- Imprecision of results
- Publication bias

Evidence Pyramid or Hierarchy of Evidence

The *Evidence Pyramid* or *Hierarchy of Evidence* (see figure 8.1) is helpful to determine which types of studies to select depending on the level of evidence required. There are many versions, although typically, in the hierarchy, the strength of the evidence diminishes further down the pyramid, and general agreement exists about the relative strength of the principal types of research (Concato, 2004; Guyatt et al., 1995). Some models place RCTs at the top of the hierarchy; however, the order noted in figure 8.1 is increasingly agreed upon, since systematic review and meta-analysis combine data from multiple RCTs, and possibly from other study types, and therefore provide the best form of evidence.

Research papers still must be appraised for quality, regardless of the level of evidence. Also, not all health issues or health interventions have been addressed through synthesized evidence reports, such as systematic reviews.

Knowledge Syntheses and Systematic Reviews

In a knowledge synthesis or systematic review (SR), a health and community practice intervention is identified and researchers examine the evidence as to whether or not this intervention works. Researchers locate, appraise, and synthesize evidence from as many relevant scientific studies as possible and summarize conclusions about effectiveness. They provide a collation of the known evidence on a given topic and identify gaps in research. Statistical methods (meta-analysis) may or may not be used to analyze and summarize the results. The Cochrane Library (www.thecochranelibrary.com) is an example of this collation.

A systematic review research paper sources and examines all the relevant studies that can possibly answer a research question for a given topic (University of York, 2015). This type of research is more than a literature review and it adheres to a strict design, thereby minimizing the chance of bias. In the SR, the goal is to search for and collect all available evidence (or as near complete recall as

Figure 8.1: Evidence Pyramid—The Hierarchy of Evidence

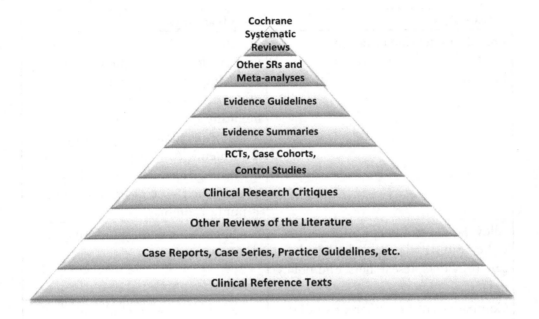

Source: Evidence-Based Practice Tools, by the Health Sciences Library, 2016, Seattle, WA: Author.

possible), including works published in peer-reviewed journals, grey literature, and unpublished research findings. A systematic approach to reviewing the literature is a more complex process than traditional literature reviews (as described in chapter 5), which are often subjective and prone to publication and language bias. The process by which studies are included or excluded is entirely transparent and is, therefore, repeatable for future updating. SRs are sometimes described as "papers that summarise other papers" ("How to Read a Paper," 1997, para. 1) and may be defined as an "overview of primary studies that used explicit reproducible methods" (Summary Points section, para. 1) in their framing of issues.

Typically, an SR will synthesize its findings from important clinical trials and may or may not include a meta-analysis. SRs are thought to constitute the best available evidence on topics in which research has been identified, selected, appraised, and synthesized in a systematic and transparent way. It is important to document search strategies in SRs to ensure reproducibility, which can be a weakness in these studies. Table 8.1 notes several advantages and disadvantages of systematic reviews.

Table 8.1: Advantages and Disadvantages of Systematic Reviews

Advantages	Disadvantages
Provide a scientific rather than subjective summarization of literature.	Systematic reviews are not the best way to address every question and many important papers are left out of the search (due to inadequate literature search or the inclusion of inadequate studies with poor quality assessment). Also, papers with more interesting results are more likely to be published—a concern referred to as publication bias.
Allow large amounts of information to be assimilated quickly by health care providers, researchers, and policy makers.	Cochrane reviews only include clinical trials.
Compare results of different studies to establish generalizability of findings and consistency of results.	Systematic reviews include an element of researcher judgment, which may also bias the review.

WHAT IS BEST PRACTICE?

"Best practices are recommendations that may evolve based on ongoing key expert experience, judgment, perspective and continued research" (Health Canada, 2006, p. 4). They are also known as "systematically developed statements of recommended practice in a specific clinical or healthy work environment area, are based on best evidence, and are designed to provide direction to practitioners and managers in their clinical and management decision making" (Field & Lohr, 1992, as cited in Registered Nurses' Association of Ontario, 2012, p. 7). A number of recognized guideline development groups, including the Registered Nurses' Association of Ontario (RNAO), have focused on bringing best evidence to practice. The Guideline International Network encompasses most of these groups, which include the Johanna Briggs Institute, the Scottish International Guideline Network, and the National Institute for Health and Clinical Excellence. While many of these groups address clinical issues relevant to nurses, largely from an interprofessional perspective, RNAO is one of the few organizations in the world that develops guidelines specifically for nurses. Indeed, the RNAO guidelines include practice recommendations tailored specifically to nursing interventions, as well as related education and policy recommendations. In addition, the RNAO maintains a major focus on guideline implementation and evaluation.

The terms *guideline*, *clinical practice guideline* (CPG), and *best practice guideline* (BPG) are often used interchangeably to describe a variety of directive tools for practice. Regardless of the source or focus, BPGs are developed and implemented to achieve one or more of the following objectives:

- To deliver effective care based on current evidence
- To resolve a problem in the clinical setting (e.g., poor management of pain)
- To achieve excellence in care delivery by meeting or exceeding quality assurance standards
- To introduce an innovation (e.g., a new test or treatment)
- To eliminate use of interventions not recognized as best practice
- To create work environments that enable clinical excellence

Guidelines are developed to provide up-to-date scientific evidence on specific areas of practice, with the goal of providing consistent and appropriate practice. Clinical practice guidelines or best practice guidelines are systematically developed statements (based on best available evidence) to assist practitioner and patient decisions about appropriate health care for specific clinical (practice) circumstances (Field & Lohr, 1992). These guidelines provide concise instructions for practice based on the best scientific evidence available. The World Health Organization (WHO) has specifically recognized the importance of ensuring that health care recommendations are informed by the best available research evidence, which is obtained through a rigorous literature identification process and composed into guidelines (World Health Organization, 2003).

Best practice guideline development is a rapidly expanding area; however, despite the increasing numbers of guidelines developed, health and community practices in general do not consistently reflect best evidence (Graham & Harrison, 2005). There are ongoing challenges in promoting full utilization of existing guidelines by practitioners, particularly if they are not effectively introduced, implemented, and supported. There is strong evidence in the literature indicating inadequate use of well-known guidelines from the field of medicine (Bero et al., 1998; Davis & Taylor-Vaisey, 1997; Oxman, Thomson,

Davis & Haynes, 1995; Thomas, McColl, Cullum, Rousseau & Soutter, 1999; Wensing, van der Weijden & Grol, 1998), as well as nursing and other health professions (Davies, Edwards, Ploeg & Virani, 2008; Higuchi, Davies, Edwards, Ploeg & Virani, 2011).

Benefits of Practice Guidelines

Practice guidelines improve the quality of clinical decisions by providing explicit, scientifically supported recommendations on the appropriateness of treatments (Woolf, Grol, Hutchinson, Eccles & Grimshaw, 1999). Guidelines assist in ensuring the consistency and efficiency of care delivered, and help to close the gap between what a practitioner does in practice and what the scientific evidence supports. Guidelines serve as a common point of reference for both prospective and retrospective clinical practice audits (Woolf et al., 1999). Gaps identified in scientific evidence alert researchers to areas of practice in need of additional research. Guidelines also assist health and community practice organizations in providing consistency of care and optimizing value for the dollar in delivery of care (Woolf et al., 1999).

Guidelines accompanied by a consumer version and/or disseminated widely to the public serve to inform patients and the public about what interprofessional practitioners should be doing. Guidelines also serve to influence public policy by drawing attention to under-recognized health problems, underserved populations, services issues, and preventive interventions (Woolf et al., 1999).

Potential Limitations of Clinical Practice Guidelines

A guideline is based on the best evidence available when the recommendation for practice is made. Unfortunately, with time, new scientific evidence may inform practitioners that the recommendation was not the best for all patients (Woolf et al., 1999). Research methodology may be flawed, and some needed research on humans cannot be conducted because of the limitations of federal government human subject research regulations.

Guidelines need to be flexible for individualized implementation based on the status of the patient and the clinical environment in which the care is delivered. Recommendations may affect decisions to provide financial support for a service. Conflicting guidelines from a variety of sources can confuse practitioners. Outdated recommendations have the potential of promoting outdated care. Lastly, guidelines that conclude a treatment or procedure may not be beneficial can be dangerous and may limit approval and/or funding for future research on the topic (Woolf et al., 1999).

HOW DO POLICIES, PROTOCOLS, AND GUIDELINES CONTRIBUTE TO EVIDENCE-INFORMED PRACTICE?

Practices are skills, interventions, techniques, and strategies used by health and community interprofessional practitioners. As one component of an intervention, an evidence-informed practice has been demonstrated to produce the desired effect for the specific case or circumstances. Evidence-informed programs are generally coordinated, multi-component interventions with demonstrated effectiveness, with the core components linked to specific outcomes. Evidence-informed programs may integrate a number of practices in a specific service delivery setting for a given population (Fixen, Naoom, Blase, Friedman & Wallace, 2005).

Several steps and components have been identified as supporting use of research in practice (Straus, Tetroe, Graham, Zwarenstein & Bhattacharyya, 2009). As introduced in chapter 1, the evidence-informed decision-making model highlights seven essential components of knowledge translation necessary for successful implementation of best practice guidelines:

1. Identify the problem: identify, review, and select knowledge tools and resources.
2. Adapt knowledge tools and resources to local context.
3. Assess barriers and facilitators to knowledge use.
4. Select, tailor, and implement interventions.
5. Monitor knowledge use.
6. Evaluate outcomes.
7. Sustain knowledge use.

These steps reflect a process that is dynamic, and at each phase preparation for the next phases and reflection on the previous phases is essential.

As you review the evidence-informed decision-making model from chapter 1 (see figure 1.1), it is evident that there are two key processes that comprise the knowledge-to-action cycle. The first is the knowledge creation process, which focuses on the identification of critical evidence and results in knowledge products. The second is the action cycle, which focuses on the application of knowledge in the practice setting. In these final chapters, we are concerned primarily with the action cycle and the application of best practice guidelines.

Before addressing the action cycle, it is important to understand that the knowledge creation portion of the model depicts the processes that are used to identify relevant knowledge (searching, appraising, synthesizing) to validate and tailor it to the specific area of practice. This is the process used in evidence-informed guideline development, in which research and other evidence is identified and synthesized into knowledge tools and products, such as practice guidelines and recommendations, clinical pathways, and decision support tools. For an example of support tool development regarding rural maternity care, refer to box 8.2.

Box 8.2: Decision Tools for Rural Maternity Care in British Columbia

Decisions about how and where to provide services for safe, effective rural maternity care must address complex and competing interests. In these areas of British Columbia, women do not always have maternity care or delivery facilities and staff available, and women in their later stages of pregnancy must leave their communities in order to give birth. Decision analysis offers tools for addressing these complexities in order to help decision makers determine the best use of resources and to appreciate the downstream effects of their decisions. The research team sought a formal decision-analysis approach that included all stakeholders. This consultation was in an effort to clarify the influences affecting rural maternity care and to develop decision-making tools for best practice. The research supported the development of an evidence-informed manual and toolkit to assist decision makers for best practice for the provision of maternity care in rural settings in Northern British Columbia.

Source: "Development of a Support Tool for Complex Decision-Making in the Provision of Rural Maternity Care," G. Hearns et al., 2010, *Healthcare Policy*, 5(3), p. 82–96.

Essentially, all guideline development methodologies incorporate a knowledge creation process, while some are more rigorous than others. Those responsible for leading policy and guideline implementation can determine the quality of knowledge products by assessing them against recognized standards for guideline development. These internationally recognized standards are available in the Appraisal of Guidelines for Research and Evaluation (AGREE II) instrument (Brouwers et al., 2010).

The action cycle of the evidence-informed decision-making model is the process by which the knowledge created is implemented, evaluated, and sustained in the practice setting. The seven phases that comprise the action cycle are based on a synthesis of evidence-informed theories that focus on the process of deliberate, systematic change in health care systems and groups (Straus et al., 2009).

The first phase of the action cycle for health and community practitioners involves identifying the problem. This identification is activated because practitioners and/or managers define a problem and then identify and review possible best practices that may help to resolve the problem. Practitioners or managers may also initiate research action when they become aware of a policy or guideline and determine whether current practice is consistent with the best practice or if practice change is necessary. This initial phase is important, as it sets the stage for the process of research in practice that is linked to ongoing quality improvement. The identified problem will be resolved through adoption of best practice, education, and policy development or revision.

The second phase—adaptation to local context (see figure 8.2)—is critical to effective knowledge translation and requires understanding of the local context and the implications of the best practice within that context so that recommendations can be adapted in ways that best fit the culture.

Figure 8.2: The Adapt Step in the Evidence-Informed Decision-Making Model

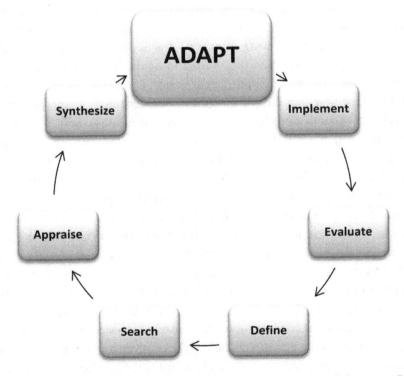

Source: Adapted from *Evidence-Informed Public Health,* by National Collaborating Centre for Methods and Tools, 2016, Hamilton, Canada: McMaster University.

Adaptation of best evidence into practice, policy, or guideline for the local setting or context requires knowledge of the evidence base underpinning the existing guideline or realities of practice. Adaptation involves establishing a process for review and selecting appropriate guidelines for use, assessing them (possibly against a quality appraisal tool such as the AGREE II quality appraisal; Brouwers et al., 2010), determining the clinical utility and feasibility for implementation of the guideline recommendations, and identifying those that are generally acceptable in the local circumstances.

Modifications to a practice, policy, or guideline may be carried out at this time by the implementation group with stakeholder input. A stakeholder is an individual, group, or organization with a vested interest in the decision to implement a best practice guideline (Baker et al., 1999). Stakeholders include all those individuals or groups who will be directly or indirectly affected by, or who can directly or indirectly affect the implementation of, a best practice guideline. A stakeholder analysis will help gather information about stakeholders for the purpose of helping the guideline implementation work with existing realities and relationships and to build on, champion, and anticipate challenges. This knowledge can help the team to determine the support, resources, and influences to determine how best to engage them for success. The aim of this phase is to select the recommendations in a transparent way that is perceived by all to reflect best evidence, address the identified problem, and fit the local circumstances.

The third phase—assess facilitators and barriers to knowledge use—moves closer to implementation of elements of the guideline, identifies barriers and facilitators to research, best practice guidelines in the environment, as well as the impacts to relevant stakeholders. Specific barriers such as lack of knowledge, attitudes, and resistance to change are critical to identify. It is important to balance against those elements that will facilitate the uptake of research in practice. Practice guidelines direct interventions, standards, protocols, education programs, and policies that are part of the daily practice of all health and community practitioners. Examples of areas in which these guidelines have been incorporated into the ongoing structures and processes in health care are highlighted in box 8.3.

While it is important that every practitioner be sure that best evidence is used, the amount of new knowledge that is produced daily makes it unrealistic to expect students and interprofessional practitioners to conduct literature reviews regularly to update their practice. As such, students and interprofessional practitioners can look to best practice guidelines to direct their practice, thus impacting the outcomes of services provided. Best practice guidelines are important as they enable practitioners to focus on the appropriate provision of care knowing they are informed by the best evidence available in the field (Ferguson-Paré, Closson & Tully, 2002).

Box 8.3: How Do Evidence-Informed Guidelines Shape Structures and Processes for Practice?

Evidence-informed guidelines can influence the following:

- Client information provided for informed decision making
- Client care plans, care maps, clinical pathways, and algorithms
- System processes and outcomes
- Vision statements, mission statements, day-to-day practice, policies, procedures, and documentation
- Learning sets and educational packages used for orientation and staff development (Krugman, 2003)

Best practice guidelines lead to policy, help to direct practice, and help to inform of appropriate standards and protocols. Brouwers et al.'s (2010) AGREE II instrument clearly identifies standards for practice guidelines and helps differentiate between a quality guideline and other practice-related documents available to practitioners in the workplace. Thousands of practice guidelines are now available and accessible to practitioners from all disciplines. These guidelines vary with respect to the level of methodological rigour used in their development, the strength of the evidence supporting recommendations, clarity, and format. Many guidelines fall short in following established methodological standards of guideline development (Brouwers et al., 2010), particularly with respect to the identification, evaluation, and synthesis of scientific evidence (Straus, Tetroe & Graham, 2009). Practitioners often need assistance in identifying and selecting guidelines that are of the highest quality and are relevant to their practice.

Practitioners strive to ensure that the approaches used in practice are producing quality outcomes and are based on the best evidence. Therefore, there are generally two ways that best practices are used to trigger a practice change. One way is that a new guideline may be made available that drives a practice review and adoption of the new guideline. Another way is that a clinical practice issue, problem, or challenge will surface that motivates a search for knowledge tools like a BPG to help determine how a new set of practices or specific practice changes can drive an effective solution. Box 8.4 highlights practice situations that indicate a knowledge-practice gap.

Box 8.4: Practice Situations Indicating a Knowledge-Practice Gap

- Stakeholders identify a practice need.
- A community partner requests assistance or collaboration with a project.
- A disaster or urgent event forces the investigation of current practices and the examination of ways to improve care.
- The government launches a new initiative or funding program.
- Particular safety issues surface.
- Quality initiatives and collected data require a response.

Once a knowledge-practice gap has been identified, it is important to look to the appropriate evidence to find the solution. Current best practice guidelines for mental health promotion are available from the Centre for Addiction and Mental Health (see box 8.5).

Major efforts have been made to improve the quality and rigour of practice guidelines in order to ensure that clinical practice will be based on the best available evidence. In keeping with the goal of using the best possible evidence in guideline development, it is equally important to use the best guidelines available. Thus, we recommend that guideline writers and adopters use a guideline evaluation instrument, such as the AGREE II instrument (Brouwers et al., 2010) or the ADAPTE methodology (ADAPTE Collaboration, 2009). Brouwers et al.'s (2010) AGREE II instrument identifies key criteria called domains that comprise a high-quality guideline and is sensitive to differences in these important domains. Once practitioners identify a knowledge-practice gap and have identified a guideline that would be useful, several steps can be carried out as part of the guideline appraisal process:

1. Identify whether or not a credible author has already conducted an up-to-date appraisal of BPGs of interest.
2. If no review is available, search available BPGs on your topic. Systematically search for related BPGs, and remember that such guidelines vary in rigour and quality. Seek help from a skilled librarian or literature search expert.
3. Access all BPGs in their entirety. A quick read often points to technical documents, monographs, or other associated literature describing

BPG development in detail and providing supporting evidence. Keep a meticulous record of guidelines accessed.

4. When many BPGs are accessed, screening criteria (e.g., inclusion and exclusion criteria) may be used to short-list guidelines of interest. Screening should ensure that guideline development was evidence informed.

Box 8.5: Research in Practice—Best Practice Guidelines for Mental Health Promotion across the Lifespan

The *Best Practice Guidelines for Mental Health Promotion Programs* are a series of online guides for interprofessional practitioners that supports practices for positive mental health across the lifespan. Current evidence-based approaches in the application of mental health promotion concepts and principles are provided in these guides. In 2016, three guides were available: one focused on older adults 55+, one on children and youth, and one on refugees. A guide with a focus on immigrants is forthcoming. Specifically, the child and youth mental health promotion resource includes information to provide health and social workers background and theory about the definitions about mental health as well as behavioural and contextual factors that influence children's mental health and social well-being, including a focus on resilience. The 10 best practice guidelines for child and youth mental health promotion interventions are provided in the document along with examples of programs that incorporate good practice. The resource also provides a worksheet that can be used by service providers to identify which guidelines can be implemented or used for future planning.

Source: Centre for Addiction and Mental Health: Health Promotion Resource Centre. (2016). *Best Practice Guidelines for Mental Health Promotion Programs*. Retrieved from www.porticonetwork.ca/web/camh-hprc/resources/best-practice-guidelines-for-mental-health-promotion-programs.

Adapting Guidelines for Practice

Guideline adaptation is an important process in the implementation of evidence-informed practice (ADAPTE Collaboration, 2009; Harrison, Graham & Fervers, 2009). Clinical practice guidelines that have been developed in one cultural or sectoral setting may be challenging to implement in another. Contextual differences may affect the suitability or feasibility of particular recommendations, even when supported by a strong body of evidence. Each local context is unique and is based on a range of factors, including organizational priorities, available resources, scopes of practice, and regional legislation. The adaptation of existing high quality practice guidelines to the local context minimizes the need to develop locally specific clinical practice guidelines and enhances the implementation of evidence-informed recommendations to the particular practice setting.

Guideline adaptation involves making decisions about the value and suitability of the knowledge presented in the source guideline to local circumstances (Graham et al., 2006). "It also encompasses those activities that the implementation team may engage in to tailor or customize the knowledge to their particular situation" (Graham et al., 2006), while maintaining the evidence-informed nature of the recommendations. The overall aim is to ensure that the guidelines and recommendations that are eventually implemented are perceived by all to address the identified problem, fit the local context, and represent the best available evidence.

REVIEW AND REFLECT

In an era of information overload and rapid production of new evidence, you can strive to bring the best evidence to your practice in a number of ways. As interprofessional practitioners or students, you must continually review the evidence in your practice policies and guidelines to see if it is current and the best available evidence. Evaluation tools can assist practitioners in determining if their policies and practices are current. Research and guidelines from other fields or other sites of practice can be adapted for your local practice, but the adaptation of research and guidelines to practice also requires careful review.

9 | HOW DO I USE RESEARCH IN PRACTICE?

"If you have knowledge, let others light their candles in it."

—Margaret Fuller

LEARNING OBJECTIVES

This chapter focuses on how to integrate skills from the preceding chapters in order to address health and community practice questions in the context of everyday practice realities. After reading this chapter and completing the practical learning activities in appendix B, you will be able to do the following:

- Discuss how evidence is applied in practice.
- Describe how you can contribute to research uptake in practice.

CHAPTER OUTLINE

- How Is Evidence Applied in Practice?
- What Is Research Uptake?
- How Can You Contribute to, and Advocate for, Best Evidence in Practice?
  - Supporting Policy or Guidelines That Implement Evidence
  - Join Forces with Other Advocates and Champions
- Review and Reflect

Despite the essential role of research, a large gap often exists between the evidence and its widespread use in practice. This *research-to-practice gap* is influenced by several factors, including limited stakeholder involvement in research, pilot project designs with little consideration for future larger scale studies, poor attempts to disseminate research findings and advocate their use, and the absence of tools and systematic efforts to replicate and expand evidence-informed interventions. Applying best evidence is one of the many aspects of appropriate health and community practice; you must let it guide your decision-making processes.

Personal knowledge, hunches, cultural sensitivity, and previous experience can never be left out of the decision-making equation. These issues should all be considered in the implementation and evaluation steps of any study. Health and community practice is both a science and an art. Research literacy is best practised when you have the combined capacities to think critically, to listen to yourself and others, and to follow your instincts, all simultaneously.

HOW IS EVIDENCE APPLIED IN PRACTICE?

You have likely witnessed the application of evidence to health and community practice on multiple levels. Policy, programs, specific projects, and individual intervention are all areas for evidence application. This leads to the question: "How do policies draw upon evidence?" Policy is a set of statements about how a particular goal (a program, project, or procedure) is to be reached. It seeks to structure and shape specific areas of practice of a large number of people. However, only a small amount of practice is dictated by policy. Policy is generally formalized in writing, whereas much practice resides in people's activities and experiences.

Policy and guidelines are not necessarily based on the tacit understanding of a group's style of practice, but rather are decisions derived from a person or body invested with authority. Those decisions are based on such things as underlying values or assumptions, wider concerns, research, study visits, consultation processes, but also on chance encounters or even politics. So, research is just one part of decision making that goes into guidelines and policies. Certainly primary concerns such as affordability, feasibility, and priorities come into play in the decision-making process regardless of the strength of research evidence (Gomm, 2000a; 2000b). Beyond these competing interests, whether evidence is informed or not, a major challenge with policy and guidelines is implementation—putting guidelines into practice.

The fourth phase of the evidence-informed decision-making model involves implementing and evaluating research for practice (e.g., tailoring interventions to the particular setting or circumstance), and requires an implementation plan that involves recipients of the service and other relevant stakeholders. This phase of implementation also includes the assessment of barriers and facilitators, the evidence on effective implementation strategies, and its relationship to monitoring, evaluating, and sustaining knowledge use. It is important for research leaders to keep in mind that knowledge transfer, as depicted in the model, is not necessarily a sequential process, as many phases need to be considered simultaneously. Refer again to the whole evidence-informed decision-making model in figure 9.1.

In addition, each phase includes resource implications, which must be identified and addressed for successful implementation of research in practice. Practical questions you may want to ask about implementation and evaluation reflect different sectors of health and community practice and are incorporated throughout the chapter. They include the following:

- Does the evidence-informed guideline apply to all areas of the organization?
- Are there specific recommendations that address known organizational needs?
- Are any recommendations already being implemented?
- Have some recommendations been partially implemented (e.g., only certain recommendations are implemented or only on some units or at certain sites)?
- Are there recommendations that must be implemented before others?
- Can any recommendations be implemented quickly?

- Are any recommendations based on higher levels of evidence than others?
- Will some recommendations take longer to implement? Are there barriers to implementation (e.g., budget, staff skill, leadership, workload, or cultural and attitudinal issues)?

Figure 9.1: Evidence-Informed Decision-Making Model Revisited

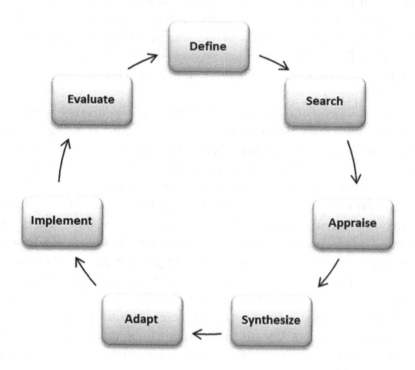

The broad issues of research uptake and specific implementation all need careful consideration as you begin to apply an evidence-informed practice in a rapidly changing age of information.

The decisions made next, based on the answers to these questions, will determine the scope of realistic implementation, as well as the resources required. Not all practice patterns will change when implementing a new guideline, and it is important to build upon existing practices and processes when committing to practice change. A total overhaul of the workplace and general upheaval is neither usually necessary nor recommended during the implementation of new best practice guidelines. With realistic and conscious awareness of the barriers and facilitators, implementation can then be directed toward reinforcing and sustaining existing best practices in the workplace. This will ultimately lead to the targeting of specific areas for practice improvement. One example of this focused work of practitioners through the evidence-informed practice process is from the recreation therapy department at Sunnybrook Health Science Centre in Toronto (see box 9.1).

Box 9.1: Research in Practice—Applying Recreation Therapy Evidence about Patient Experience in Practice

The recreation therapy department at Sunnybrook Health Science Centre in Toronto implemented best practice care through the use of standardized tools for functional assessments of clients' abilities as well as leisure inventories of their activities. Through reflection and research supported by leaders in the institution, these practices were discovered not to be meaningful to the clients they were serving—discoveries that were eye-opening! Further research, in partnership with the University of Waterloo Recreation and Leisure Studies program, was initiated and examined several key domains of practice: (1) Personal leisure profiles, (2) being with the person (in recreational therapy), (3) meaningful experiences in leisure, (4) interpretation of "community" by residents (veterans in long-term care) as part of their leisure, (5) creation of the quality indicators, (6) resident-focused documentation, and (7) experience and meaning for residents in recreation therapy. Capturing the experience of care, understanding what truly matters, and adapting the research for practice required a renegotiation of how recreation therapy needs/preferences were assessed, delivered, and evaluated. For instance, rather than completing an assessment for clients upon their admission to the service, clients are now asked to engage in a conversation with the recreation therapy department about their previous and current leisure interests and the meaning that these hold. The purpose of this is not only to learn about their interest in leisure activities, but to also learn about each client as a person and to begin to develop a therapeutic relationship. Consequently, the planning of services can incorporate clients' hopes and dreams. The conclusion of the program/activity now marks an opportunity for reflection. Periodically, clients are also asked to complete an evaluation that requests them to describe what quality indicators were met through their participation. Importantly, these results are then correlated with those identified by the recreation therapist to assess for congruence. If the outcomes do not align with the objectives of the program, then the program is reviewed and changes are made to make it more suitable for them. Through this research process, the department leaders and practitioners have moved from critical reflection to a willingness to investigate alternatives to the status quo, and toward a commitment to adapting evidence into their service provision.

Sources: Briscoe, C.L. (2012). *Narrative Exploration of Therapeutic Relationships in Recreation Therapy Through a Self-Reflective Case Review Process.* Master of Arts (Recreation and Leisure Studies) Thesis. University of Waterloo; Saint Elizabeth Person and Family Centred Care Institute. (2016). *Promising Practice 3—Quality Indicators in Recreational Therapy.* Retrieved from www.saintelizabeth.com/Services-and-Programs/PFCC-Institute/Promising-Practices.aspx.

WHAT IS RESEARCH UPTAKE?

The uptake of research for practice is what happens as ideas are transferred between people—not papers. The process of implementation of research is indeed complex; as a result, the average length of the time gap from research discovery to implementation is 17 years (Morris, Wooding & Grant, 2011).

Research results flow in a number of different directions, including toward practitioners, policy makers, and the public. Research results also take time to be accepted and verified, and researchers often first share them with other researchers. This usually occurs at research conferences or in academic journal articles that may only be read by other academics. Ideas take time to develop and researchers need to share them with their peers first. As they do so, preliminary ideas, findings, research methods, and tools spread in several directions. In this way, when researchers share results in many different formats (e.g., technical, popular media, reports, etc.), their work can appeal to different audiences. How this uptake happens, and the steps to understanding how research will flow, takes a number of forms (Graham & Harrison, 2005).

Research uptake is described as comprising four related activities: stakeholder engagement, capacity building (to support both supply of and demand for research evidence), communication, and monitoring and evaluation of uptake (Graham & Harrison, 2005). Table 9.1 illustrates the activities and steps. Each of these activities within research uptake is discussed in more detail below.

Table 9.1: Research Uptake Activities

Stakeholder Engagement	Capacity Building	Communication	Monitoring and Evaluation
• Mapping of stakeholders • Tailoring research to meet user needs • Ongoing stakeholder–researcher connection • Interactive discussion of research results	• Assess internal and external capacity for research and use • Continually monitoring capacity and building strategy accordingly • Design and implement capacity-building activities	• Design initial communication strategy • Rigorous synthesis of research • Package and disseminate emerging results • Adapt communication strategy with emerging results	• Design research uptake objectives and align with organizational or program objectives • Gain data and understanding of uptake (or lack thereof) • Adapt research, capacity building, and communication based on uptake discoveries

The uptake of research is rarely about the research findings alone, no matter how strong or weak the findings may be. That said, the quality of the research itself is an important element and is why your literacy and capacity to perform critical appraisal is so important. If the findings were all stakeholders cared about, then research outputs would not be more than a few paragraphs or bullet points long. Not all the research being used by practitioners, organizations, policy makers, and others is strong enough to warrant implementation, however. The systematic scrutiny of research and collection of research takes time, which is one reason why the length of time from research discoveries to uptake can be so very long.

Alongside the steps of quality assessment and synthesis of evidence, there are many concerns that will determine uptake. Researchers do not control political agendas, and they do not control fluctuations (e.g., the economy, social conflicts, natural disasters, technological change, etc.) that may affect the prompt transfer of new research findings.

Uptake is often equated with instituting what the paper or study recommends. Even with all the right circumstances, in terms of stakeholder engagement, it is unlikely that our health and community practice organizations will achieve more than just a bit of uptake. At any one time, research can offer alternative courses of action and assess their effects, but the research and the researchers themselves do not ultimately take the actions for evidence-informed decision making. As an everyday example, research has shown that consumption of alcohol increases the risk for breast cancer (Hamajima, Hirose, Tajima, Rohan, Calle, Heath Jr., et al., 2002), but many still choose to drink. While the research is known and used, it is considered alongside other evidence (e.g., research that also indicates one drink of red wine decreases risk of heart attack, anecdotal evidence such as "my aunt drank wine every day and lived to 97 in perfect health," and other values). However, the choice and specific recommendations and actions are yours to take—as interprofessional practitioners, students, managers, leaders, policy makers, and those working in all areas of health and community practice. Good uptake happens when good ideas, practices, and people are incorporated into a shared decision-making process. What we desire is good decision-making capacity and involvement with the end users of research, not just good evidence-informed decisions. The critical thinking and decision-making capacity you will develop as a student and interprofessional practitioner will continually be tested in this way, and will continue to challenge you throughout your career. Therefore, to really understand and support research uptake, you need to care about and understand your clients' and community's needs, as well as the needs of stakeholders.

HOW CAN YOU CONTRIBUTE TO, AND ADVOCATE FOR, BEST EVIDENCE IN PRACTICE?

Supporting Policy or Guidelines That Implement Evidence

Supporting best practice guidelines and policies by drawing on recommendations from strong evidence will go a long way to utilizing appropriate evidence-informed practice. New and evidence-informed practices can often be implemented without policy changes, but policy changes are often crucial for the large-scale implementation and support of new practices. Most new practices require multiple levels of implementation to become established and adopted in sustainable ways.

Join Forces with Other Advocates and Champions

There is strength in numbers—being part of a team of champions for a desired change always lends strength to bringing about evidence-informed practice changes. Joining forces with other champions from different spheres of influence will build the strength further. For example, when advocating for a community health issue, consider engaging a political leader, a health sector leader, other interprofessional practitioners, students, and most definitely community members. Having multiple champions can help facilitate and institutionalize change at multiple levels. Having champions who may have particular influence in a community (a local spokesperson, celebrity, or particularly influential insider) may also be helpful.

You may want to seek financial support and provide guidance to champions of a research cause, so that the commitment and consistency will be sustained. Providing administrative, secretarial, or financial support (such as a stipend, travel expenses, or refreshments at meetings) for champions as well as talking points or other materials to implement advocacy activities can also support implementation (Wilson, Brady & Lesesne, 2011). Performance support tools (e.g., a checklist) that can be used to present a detailed policy or guideline in a concise and easy-to-follow format are other useful instruments to aid in the implementation of evidence-informed decisions. Research assistants help with memory recall for practitioners by performing complicated or repetitive tasks and outlining the minimum expected steps in a complex process (Edson, Koniz-Booher, Boucar, et al., 2002). Consider these recommendations for aids to evidence-informed guideline checklists, job aids, or other infographics:

- Involve those who will use the job aid in creating it, including content review and field testing.
- Consider the language, education, and literacy levels of those who will use the job aid.
- Create a simple format so the job aid is easy to follow.
- As appropriate, consider using illustrations or diagrams, including decision-making algorithms.
- Consider the job aid's portability if practitioners travel frequently between settings. If the job aid is too heavy or cumbersome, it will not be used.
- Develop an addendum to the job aid with information explaining the evidence, policies, and guidelines on which the job aid is based.
- Plan for how practitioners will learn to use job aids. Actively disseminate job aids—through the training and supervision of providers—to improve outcomes.
- As guidelines change, update job aids and retrain providers, highlighting the changes that have been made.

Go to activity 9.1 in appendix B to locate and review infographics and job aids of interest for your practice. As you work to bring evidence to your practice in meaningful ways, be curious, committed, and patient! Certain goals, especially those linked to policy change, may require a longer duration of advocacy than others.

REVIEW AND REFLECT

In conclusion, research uptake can be many things, and it depends on you, professional and individual choices, realities of individuals' health and social determinants of health, your community practice organization's strategy and objectives, as well as the context in which the organization works. Research uptake involves many creative strategies, tools, and technologies. It must begin with basic research literacy and be supported by a solid research appraisal.

FURTHER RESOURCES AND LINKS

> "What is research but a blind date with knowledge."
>
> —William Henry

The preceding chapters have introduced you to research language that can inform your search and reading of research in health and community practice, as well as improve your understanding, interpretation, and use of it. Like with any new language, if you don't speak and practice your new skills, they quickly slip away! In the following pages, you will find additional reference material to review and work with in order to sustain and deepen your understanding of previous lessons. We also include links to many useful tutorials and additional learning modules, followed by an expansive glossary of research terms employed in the textbook (and beyond); practice exam questions; and, finally, learning activities so you can continue to immerse yourself in this language. If research is "a blind date with knowledge," your literacy and growth in this area is a long-term relationship!

1. The Cochrane Collaboration
The Cochrane Collaboration is an independent global network of over 30,000 health care practitioners, researchers, patient advocates, and others. Cochrane works to turn the evidence generated through research into useful information for making everyday decisions about health (www.cochrane.org/about-us). The PICO Question Tutorial is available at the University of Oxford website's Cochrane

Library Tutorial. The tutorial (and other resources at the university website) offers support in understanding ways to formulate an answerable question in pursuit of evidence for practice.

http://learntech.physiol.ox.ac.uk/cochrane_tutorial/cochlibd0e84.php

2. Critical Appraisal Skills Programme (CASP)

The Critical Appraisal Skills Programme (CASP) is part of Better Value Healthcare, a training organization led by Professor Sir Muir Gray, and based in Oxford. The program has developed workshops and tools for critical appraisal covering a wide range of research. It has also developed finding the evidence workshops, and interactive and e-learning resources. The philosophy of CASP is about sharing knowledge and understanding, working in ways that are non-hierarchical and multidisciplinary, and using problem-based approaches. This ensures that it is accessible and has practical day-to-day application.

www.casp-uk.net/

3. Interagency Panel on Research Ethics (Government of Canada)

The Interagency Panel on Research Ethics in Canada has developed an online learning experience that features interactive and multidisciplinary examples to learn the core principles related to research ethics review. It is designed primarily for those conducting research or reviewing the ethical concerns related to human subject involvement in research, though anyone may take this course and print their own certificate of completion.

www.pre.ethics.gc.ca/eng/education/tutorial-didacticiel/

4. The Joanna Briggs Institute

The Joanna Briggs Institute (JBI) is the international not-for-profit research and development centre within the Faculty of Health Sciences at the University of Adelaide, South Australia. The institute collaborates internationally with over 70 entities across the world. The institute and its collaborating entities promote and support the synthesis, transfer, and utilization of evidence through identifying feasible, appropriate, meaningful, and effective health care practices to assist in the improvement of health care outcomes globally.

http://joannabriggs.org/index.html

5. McMaster University

McMaster's Faculty of Health Sciences places a strong emphasis on evidence-based practice (EBP). On this page, you will learn about the core concepts of EBP and be directed to additional resources for deepening your knowledge and improving your evidence-based skills.

http://hsl.mcmaster.libguides.com/c.php?g=306765&p=2044668

6. National Collaborating Centre for Methods and Tools (NCCMT)

The National Collaborating Centre for Methods and Tools is one of six National Collaborating Centres for Public Health in Canada. NCCMT provides leadership and expertise in evidence-informed decision making to Canadian public health organizations. The NCCMT provides numerous free learning resources, online educational tutorials, and reference materials concerned with evidence-informed practice and research appraisal and literacy.

www.nccmt.ca

7. National Institute for Health and Care Excellence (NICE)

NICE's role is to improve outcomes for people using the United Kingdom's National Health Service and other public health and social care services. They do this through the following initiatives:

- Producing evidence-based guidance and advice for health, public health and social care practitioners.
- Developing quality standards and performance metrics for those providing and commissioning health, public health, and social care services.
- Providing a range of information services for commissioners, practitioners, and managers across the spectrum of health and social care.

www.nice.org.uk

8. Practice and Research Together (PART)

PART is a Canadian membership-based research utilization initiative. PART's core function is to distill and disseminate practice-relevant research findings to child welfare practitioners including front-line practitioners, senior leaders, and caregivers. PART promotes evidence-informed practice through a variety of innovative program components, including PARTicle literature reviews, webinars, large scale conferences, practice guidebooks, and electronic access to research and academic journals. PART also provides support to individual member agencies as they implement evidence-informed practice.

www.partcanada.org/about-part

9. Research in Practice (RIP)
RIP aims to bridge the gaps among research, practice, and service users' lived experiences to improve practice and ultimately outcomes for children and families. Numerous publications, training materials, and supports for evidence-informed practice are available at this link: www.rip.org.uk. Another arm of the organization holds similar objectives and provides numerous resources and best practices supports for health and community practice for adults: www.ripfa.org.uk.

GLOSSARY

Absolute risk: The actual probability or likelihood that an event will occur itself is often referred to as the *absolute risk*. The higher the absolute risk is, the more likely it is that the something will happen—although it still is not guaranteed to take place. This risk is understood by dividing the number of events (good or bad) in treated or control groups by the number of people in that group.

Abstract: A brief, objective summary of the essential content of a book, article, speech, report, dissertation, or other work that presents the main points in the same order as the original but has no independent literary value. In a scholarly journal article, the abstract follows the title and the name(s) of the author(s) and precedes the text. In an entry in a printed indexing and abstracting service or bibliographic database, the abstract accompanies the citation.

Analysis of variance (ANOVA): A statistical test for comparing mean differences in three or more groups by comparing variability among groups.

Anthropology: The study of humans and human behaviours.

Application of knowledge: The iterative process by which knowledge is put into practice.

Appraise: The process of assessing the quality of study methods in order to determine if findings are trustworthy, meaningful, and relevant to your situation.

Association: A potential causal connection between two variables.

Authority: The knowledge and experience that qualifies a person to write or speak as an expert on a given subject. In the academic community, authority is based on credentials, previously published works on the subject, institutional affiliation, awards, imprint, reviews, patterns of citation, etc.

Autonomy: The ability to make choices for oneself.

Average: The common name of the arithmetic *mean*, which is the sum of all the observations in a data set divided by the number of observations.

Behavioural bias: Bias that occurs when people within a study behave in a given manner because of some underlying reason that usually affects all similar individuals.

Beneficence: The ethical principle of doing good.

Best practice guideline (BPG): Practice recommendations that are usually based on a rigorous review of many studies by experts on the topic. In reference to clinical practice issues, also called *best practice guideline*.

Bias: In the context of research, anything in the design or undertaking of a study that causes an untruth to occur in the study potentially affecting the outcome of the study. See also *measurement bias*, *recall bias*, *response bias*, and *selection bias*.

Bibliography: In the context of scholarly publication, a list of references to sources cited in the text of an article or book, or suggested by the author for further reading; it is usually given at the end of the work.

Blinding: The process of hiding from either the participant (single blind) or both the participant and the researchers (double blind) to which arm of a study (usually a randomized controlled trial) a participant is allocated. Also known as masking.

Bracketing: A phenomenological research process to identify and suspend any of the researcher's preconceived notions about the topic.

Broader term: In a hierarchical classification system, a subject heading or descriptor that includes another term as a subclass (for example, "Libraries" listed as a broader term under "School libraries"). In some indexing systems, a subject heading or descriptor may have more than one broader term (for example, "Documentation" and "Library science" under "Cataloguing").

Capacity development: The development of knowledge, skills, and attitudes among individuals and groups of people. It also involves the creation of structures, resources, policies, and procedures in organizations and networks to sustain and achieve relevant goals, cope with complexity, and innovate.

Case-control study: A design that matches similar types of patients who receive a treatment (i.e., cases) with patients who do not receive the treatment (i.e., controls). A case-control study involves identifying people who have the outcome of interest (cases) and control patients without the same outcome, and looking to see if they had the exposure of interest.

Case report: A study reporting observations on a single individual.

Case series: A report on a series of patients with an outcome of interest with no comparison group.

Case study: A research design that focuses in depth on specific (often small) populations or well-defined events that are bounded by time.

Causality: A relationship of cause and effect that meets (at a minimum) the following three conditions: a strong relationship between the proposed cause and effect; the proposed cause precedes the effect in time; and the proposed cause must be present whenever the effect occurs.

Causation: Studies that consider risk factors (exposure) for certain diseases/problems/conditions (outcomes)—for instance, the effect of patient characteristics (exposure) on the development of pressure ulcers (outcome). Also referred to as "etiology" or "aetiology."

Cause: In a study of the relationships of variables, the cause is the agency or event that connects and creates the change in another process (the effect). It is measured as the independent variable.

Central tendency: Measures of the centre of the scores in a given data set. These may also be called a centre or location of the distribution. The most common measures of central tendency are the arithmetic mean, the median, and the mode.

Chi-square test (x^2): A statistical test to assess differences (and to identify if there is any statistically significant difference) in proportions using data that come from one or more categories.

Citation: A reference that lists the bibliographic details of the material paraphrased, mentioned, or quoted in your research. The reference provides information such as title, author, journal title, volume, issue, publisher, and date of publication so as to identify the specific resource used.

Clinical practice guideline: An evidence-informed recommendation, usually based on a rigorous review of many studies by experts on a topic, for care that should be accompanied by practitioner judgment and experience, as well as patient preferences.

Clinical relevance: How well a study proposal, or the results, addresses a meaningful issue related to practice.

Clinical significance: Assesses whether the size of the effect of an intervention is big enough to justify the investment required for its implementation. Assessing clinical significance takes into account factors such as the size of a treatment effect, importance of the problem being addressed, other potential outcomes of the intervention, and cost of implementation.

Cluster randomized controlled trial: Randomization by cluster or group to an experimental intervention or a control group.

Cochrane Collaboration: An international organization for the development and updating of systematic reviews on health care effectiveness topics.

Cohort study: A design referred to as an observational study that monitors a defined group (cohort) or subgroups (cohorts) over time. It involves the identification of two groups (cohorts) of patients, one that did receive the exposure of interest, and one that did not, and follows these cohorts forward for the outcome of interest.

Collaboration: A process of interaction where people (e.g., interprofessional practitioners) work together to achieve desired outcomes.

Common knowledge: Something that is generally known. Information that is *not* of a specialist or arcane nature or that requires specific study or training.

Community of practice: Voluntary, flexible networks of people with a common interest that learn, share knowledge, and develop expertise on an issue.

Comparison group: Participants in a study who receive the standard of care or conventional treatment instead of the experimental treatment (intervention).

Concept: An abstract idea formed by examining specific instances. It cannot be measured directly and is based on observations of certain behaviours or characteristics (e.g., grief).

Conceptual model or framework: A term that refers to how variables are expected to relate to each other and why (e.g., variables related to CAM use). At a higher level of abstraction, it may be defined as concepts that are interrelated by virtue of their relevance to a common theme (e.g., psychological and social factors related to the decision-making process).

Confidence interval (CI): The likely range of the true value of interest (e.g., the effect of an intervention or treatment). The CI is usually reported as "95% CI," which means that 95 percent of the time the true value (effect) for the population lies within the given range of values.

Confidence level: This level tells you how sure you can be about a given result. For example, a 0% confidence level means you have **no faith at all** that if you repeated the test that you would get the same results. A 100% confidence level means there is **no doubt at all** that if you repeated the test you would get the same results. Practically, a 100% confidence level does not exist in statistics, unless an entire population was studied—and even then you probably couldn't be 100 percent sure the test was not influenced by some kind of error or bias.

Confirmability: A component of qualitative validity, confirmability refers to the degree to which the results could be confirmed or corroborated by others.

Conflict of interest: The incompatibility of two or more duties, responsibilities, or interests (personal or professional) of an individual or institution as they relate to the ethical conduct of research, such that one cannot be fulfilled without compromising another.

Confounder: A factor that is associated with both an intervention (or exposure) and an outcome of interest. For example, if people in the experimental group of a controlled trial are younger than those in the control group, it will be difficult to decide whether a lower risk of death in one group is due to the intervention or the difference in age. Age is then said to be a confounder, or a confounding variable. Confounding is a major concern in non-randomized studies, given there is greater chance that confounders will not be equally distributed among groups.

Confounding: Confounding occurs when researchers do not account for alternative explanations for an outcome in a study. Confounding variables are always independently associated with both the exposure and the measured outcome. For example, an increased risk of cancer of the pancreas is associated with both smoking and coffee drinking, and smokers tend to drink more coffee than non-smokers.

Constant comparison: A grounded theory analysis technique to clarify a developing theory by comparing data as they are collected with previously collected data.

Construct: A highly abstract concept that cannot be measured directly. Such a concept is invented (constructed) by researchers for the purposes of research. Constructs are measured using multiple items that in combination assess their meaning. Examples of constructs are locus of control, self-efficacy, and CAM. The terms *concept* and *construct* are often used interchangeably as they are very close in meaning.

Construct validity: The degree to which an instrument measures the construct under investigation. There are various ways to assess construct validity; however, they are all based on the logical analysis of hypothesized relationships between constructs: If constructs A and B are related, then instruments for A and B should also be related. Or if C and D are instruments to measure the same construct, then instruments C and D should be related. Convergent validity and discriminant validity are subtypes of construct validity. *Convergent validity* is the degree to which measures of constructs that theoretically should be related to each other are, in fact, observed to be related to each other (i.e., they converge). *Discriminant validity* is the degree to which measures of constructs that theoretically should not be related to each other are, in fact, observed to not be related to each other (i.e., they discriminate).

Content validity: The degree to which an instrument is consistent with (1) the known literature about the construct that the instrument attempts to measure, and (2) the opinion of experts who have done work in the field.

Continuing education: Planned educational activities intended to further the education and training of specific health professionals through the enhancement of practice, education, administration, and research.

Continuing professional development: The process by which health professionals keep updated to meet the needs of patients, health services, and their own professional development. It includes the continuous acquisition of new knowledge, skills, and attitudes to enable competent practices.

Control group: The group of a randomized controlled trial to which the intervention under study is not applied. People in this group are otherwise treated in the same way as people in the intervention group. This allows the researchers to be sure that the intervention under study *causes* the outcome they are measuring.

Convenience sample: A sample taken from a set of individuals who are easily accessed.

Correlation: An apparent association (or mutual relation) between two variables. A *positive correlation* occurs in situations when an increase or decrease in the independent variable occurs in parallel with a similar increase or decrease in the dependent variable. A *negative correlation* occurs when a rise in the value of the independent variable occurs alongside a decrease in one variable, in concert with a decrease in the other variable.

Correlation design: A design that examines the statistical interrelationships among variables. It is also known as *correlational research*.

Course-based research activities: Assignments for students within the context of a course that meet the definition of research but are not conducted for a research purpose. The intent of these activities is usually to give students experience in the conducting research (e.g., surveying other students outside of class, or observing people at a concert) and to provide material for a course-related project. They are also known as *course-related research activities*.

CRAAP test: A mnemonic strategy for evaluating information sources: C = Currency, R = Relevance, A = Authority, A = Accuracy, P = Purpose.

Credible (credibility): Believable. A term used in qualitative research referring to the ability of a study to reveal the truth, and the probability that the study's methods will produce plausible findings.

Criterion validity: Multiple measures of the same concept: one is compared to a second instrument that measures the same concept. This second instrument is the criterion by which the validity of the new instrument is assessed. It should be a measure of the target construct that is widely accepted as a valid measure of that construct (a criterion measure). Criterion validity is divided into two subtypes: concurrent validity and predictive validity. *Concurrent validity* is a type of criterion validity that assesses the degree to which the scores of a measure relate to the score(s) of a criterion measure, when the two scores are assessed concurrently (for example, the relationship between behavioural ratings from the staff in a mental institution regarding readiness for discharge and a formal test that assesses readiness for discharge). *Predictive validity* is a type of criterion validity that assesses if scores on a new instrument can predict future standing, status, or performance (for example, whether grades can predict academic success, or a test to assess if readiness for discharge can predict re-hospitalization).

Critical appraisal: The process of systematically examining research to judge its trustworthiness, value, and relevance in a particular context.

Critical theory: A social theory oriented to the critique of dominant ideas with the intent to create social and cultural change.

Cross-sectional study: A type of observational study that analyzes data collected from a population, or a representative subset, at a specific point in time. Cross-sectional studies are conducted in order to determine the relationship between disease (or other health related states) and other variables of interest.

Data: The actual words or measurements gathered for a study in order to test a hypothesis or examine a problem or question.

Database: A large, regularly updated file of digitized information (bibliographic records, abstracts, full-text documents, directory entries, images, statistics, etc.) related to a specific subject or field, consisting of records of uniform format organized for ease and speed of search and retrieval and managed with the aid of database management system (DBMS) software. Content is created by the database producer (for example, the American Psychological Association), which usually publishes a print version (psychological abstracts) and leases the content to one or more database vendors (EBSCO, OCLC, etc.) that provide electronic access to the data after it has been converted to machine-readable form (PsycINFO), usually on CD-ROM or online via the Internet, using proprietary search software. Most databases used in libraries are catalogues, periodical indexes, abstracting services, and full-text reference resources leased annually under licensing agreements that limit access to registered borrowers and library staff.

Data saturation: A point in qualitative studies when there are no new ideas noted in the data analysis and it is noted that saturation of themes and categories has occurred.

Decision makers: A term for people who work in the public health field, ranging from frontline community health providers (e.g., public health nurses, environmental health inspectors, dental hygienists, health promoters, etc.) to administrators (e.g., medical officers of health, program managers) and policy makers in provincial and federal government.

Deductive approach: A quantitative approach applying known facts or theory. This is an approach to research that sets out to prove an existing idea or hypothesis. The research sets out to explore the truthfulness of the original idea.

Dependability: A component of qualitative validity, dependability refers to the concept of consistency within a study, and whether the process of research is logical and clearly documented, particularly as it relates to the chosen method and decisions made by the researchers.

Dependent variable (DV): The outcome variable of the study that occurs as a result of the independent variable having occurred (also called the outcome).

Descriptive phenomenology: The study of the essence of being with or without interpretation; that is, phenomenology may literally just describe the phenomenon of interest or may offer an interpretive lens.

Descriptive statistics: Statistics used to describe the frequencies and patterns of numbers within a data set.

Descriptive study: A study that describes characteristics of a sample of individuals. Unlike an experimental study, the investigators do not actively intervene to test a hypothesis, but rather simply describe the health status or characteristics of a sample from a defined population. Descriptive studies include case reports, case series, qualitative studies, and surveys (cross-sectional studies).

Directly measurable outcomes: Outcomes that do not require a standardized, pre-tested measuring instrument to be assessed. Some examples are cost, some biological markers, and number of days of work lost.

Dissemination: Dissemination involves identifying the appropriate audience, and tailoring the message and medium to the audience. Dissemination activities can include such things as summary/briefings to stakeholders, educational sessions with patients, practitioners, and policy makers, engagement of knowledge users in developing and executing dissemination/implementation plan, tools creation, and media engagement.

Ecological study: A kind of epidemiological study in which the unit of analysis is a population or community (defined in various ways) rather than an individual. For instance, an ecological study may look at the association between smoking and lung cancer deaths in different countries. Disease rates and exposures are measured in each of a series of populations and their relation is examined. Often the information about disease and exposure is abstracted from published statistics and therefore does not require expensive or time-consuming data collection.

Economic or decision analyses: A study that uses explicit, quantitative methods (often based on economic outcomes) to analyze decisions (i.e., on intervention choices, etc.) under conditions of uncertainty.

Effect: The trend or result measured in a research study that specifically explores causal relationships. It is understood as the dependent variable; that is, it depends on the cause (the independent variable) to create the effect. For example, in research on the relationship of drinking alcohol on reading comprehension, reading comprehension would be considered the effect.

Effectiveness [study]: A study designed to reflect ordinary, everyday conditions, usually conducted after successful results of an efficacy study.

Effect size: The strength of a relationship between two variables or an estimate of the impact of an intervention.

Efficacy [study]: A study designed with highly controlled conditions reflecting an ideal situation.

Emergent design: A qualitative research design that is not fixed and may change during the process of data collection in order to learn more about the problem or issue from the participants.

Emic: Taking the insider view—seeing the world from someone else's point of view.

Empirical: The notion of discovering new things using the senses or, in the case of research, different methods.

Empirical research (evidence): Knowledge obtained by means of direct and indirect observation or experience epidemiology (for example, the study of diseases and their treatments from a population perspective).

Epidemiology: The study of patterns of disease.

Epistemology: The philosophy of knowledge.

Equivalence studies: Comparative studies that compare a new treatment to the current best treatment rather than a placebo.

Ethics: A system of moral values, or the way people distinguish right from wrong. Research ethics are specifically concerned with analysis of ethical issues that arise when people are involved as participants in research.

Ethnographic research: Research using a qualitative method, based in anthropology, that focuses on a group's culture to learn its worldview. Data collection approaches include participant observation, in-depth interviews, and fieldwork.

Etic: The outsider's view of something.

Evaluate/evaluation research: Efforts aimed at determining, as systematically and objectively as possible, the relevance, effectiveness, and impact of health and other community activities in relation to objectives.

Evidence: Information or facts from a variety of both qualitative and quantitative sources that are systematically obtained—i.e., obtained in a way that is replicable, observable, credible, verifiable, or basically supportable.

Evidence-informed decision making: Recognizes that important evidence comes from a variety of sources: community health issues and local context; public health resources; community and political climate; and the best available research findings. Decision makers must draw on their explicit and tacit public health knowledge and expertise to incorporate all the relevant factors into the final decision, conclusion, or recommendation.

Evidence-informed practice model: Practice decisions based on reliable and valid research and other systematic information (that should take into account practitioner experience and judgment and patient preferences).

Experimental: A way of testing a hypothesis through comparison.

Experimental group: Participants in a study who receive the experimental treatment or intervention.

Experimental variable: The intervention or treatment being manipulated. It is also called the *independent variable*.

Explicit (propositional) knowledge: Formal and systematic, explicit knowledge is that which can be expressed in words and numbers, and can be easily communicated and shared.

Exposure: Contact with something that influences the development of an outcome or improves the outcome for a person (e.g., exposure to something that causes an increased risk for developing a disease or, in people who already have the disease, reaching a particular endpoint).

External validity: The extent to which the research results can be generalized or applied to other settings or samples.

Extraneous variable: A variable that confounds (confuses) the relationship between the independent and dependent variables.

Factor analysis: A statistical approach to find the most important combination of dependent variables to form an outcome measure, where there are multiple dependent variables.

Feminist theory: Focuses on issues of oppression particularly related to gender and how these issues and experiences have influenced women *and* men socially and historically. It is typically concerned with anti-oppressive methods.

Field notes: The notes taken in a qualitative research setting (the field) about observations made and interpretations of them.

Focus group: A group of individuals interviewed together on a topic common to all of them.

Full-text: Documents available online that are complete and entire. An electronic resource that provides the entire text of a single work (e.g., Britannica Online) or articles published in one or more journals, magazines, and newspapers. For example, a bibliographic database that provides the complete text of a significant proportion of the works indexed, in addition to the bibliographic citation and (in many cases) an abstract of the content. (Also full text.)

Generalize (generalizability): Refers to the ability of the findings of a study to be extrapolated to the wider population.

Gold standard: The best available measure of a study variable (the measure incurring the least error).

Government information: Reports, articles, and statistics provided by provincial and federal governments (e.g., Statistics Canada).

Grounded theory: Qualitative research in which the ultimate intent is to develop theory from data that are derived (grounded) from real-world examples.

Harm: Adverse consequences of exposure to a stimulus.

Hawthorne effect: A result that occurs when people respond in the manner in which they believe they should when confronted by a researcher asking questions. The Hawthorne effect can bias a study.

Health: According to the World Health Organization, a state of complete physical, mental, and social well-being and not merely the absence of disease or infirmity.

Health outcome domains: Groupings of different types of health outcomes that are intended to capture changes in a person's health status, quality of life, level of function, and sense of well-being that can be attributed to an intervention.

Hermeneutics: The interpretation and understanding of language.

Historical research: An investigation for patterns and trends among past events and their relevancy to the present.

Homogeneous: The same.

Homogeneous sampling: A sampling method used in qualitative research whereby researchers decide at the beginning of the study to select participants who can provide similar stories or narratives on a phenomenon. Often selection is based on shared demographics or characteristics.

Hypothesis: A statement that predicts relationships between variables. An idea that quantitative research sets out to prove. (Plural is *hypotheses*.)

Impact factor: This is a score that rates the frequency with which the average article in a journal has been cited, typically in a particular year or over five years. Higher scores reflect increased citation frequency and use by subsequent authors.

Impracticable: Incapable of being put into practice due to degree of hardship or onerousness that jeopardizes the conduct of the research—it does not mean mere inconvenience.

Incidence: The number of new instances of an event (e.g., an illness) in a given period of time.

Independent variable (IV): The causal variable in a study, which may be manipulated during a study (also called the *exposure*).

Indirectly measurable health outcomes: Outcomes that measure a construct and thus require a standardized, pre-tested, often multidimensional instrument to be assessed in a valid manner. Some examples are stress, well-being, power, and adjustment.

Inductive approach: The qualitative research process of working from specific observations and data to general conclusions.

Inferential statistics: Statistics that are used to draw conclusions about the level of association between two or more variables within a study.

Information literacy: Competence in locating, evaluating, and effectively using needed information.

Information sources: Each item of information is created in context to its originator's purpose, whether it was to inform, entertain, or educate; the originator (or source) of that information in this way may be a peer-reviewed and academic journal, an academic popular communication magazine, a journalistic source, and so on.

Informed consent: An ethical practice and research process whereby subjects must know enough about the research to decide whether to participate, and they must agree to take part voluntarily.

Integrated knowledge translation (IKT): Process that involves engaging and integrating those who will need to act on the findings, the knowledge users, into the research process.

Integrative review: A review of the literature that assimilates the results of research studies by comparing and contrasting them in order to describe the state of knowledge. It may include quantitative and qualitative research studies.

Interactionalist: A philosophical approach that is concerned with how individuals view the world and how they operate in it.

Internal consistency: The degree of correlation among items on a multi-item outcome measure instrument.

Internal validity: The extent to which a study design and methodology produce valid, accurate results, and uncontrolled or extraneous factors are not responsible for the outcomes.

Interpretability: The degree to which one can assign easily understood meaning to an instrument's score (e.g., what a score of 70 means about a person's cognitive functioning on a scale that measures cognitive ability in a range from 0 to 100).

Interpretative description: Qualitative data analysis that attempts to apply an interpretation or understanding to the data collected from the research participants.

Inter-rater reliability: The degree to which two people (raters) working independently, using the same research tool (to rate or gather information) at the same time, get similar results.

Intervention: The aspect of interest in experimental and observational studies. Interventions can be therapeutic (e.g., different wound dressings), preventative (e.g., influenza vaccination), and diagnostic (e.g., measurement of blood pressure), targeted at individuals, groups, organizations, communities, or health systems.

Intervention research: Generally an approach to quantitative research when an intentional intervention is applied to a research subject in order to measure the effect of the intervention (may also involve some aspects of qualitative research).

Journal: A publication with a set title, issued at regular and stated intervals (e.g., quarterly), which is intended to continue publication for an indefinite period into the future. A journal contains documents, usually articles, written by different authors. The contents of any specific issue of a given journal will vary; however, most journals publish documents that deal with a particular academic discipline, subject, or area of research (for example, *Journal of Air Transportation* or *International Journal of Educational Research*). Journals, and especially scholarly journals, contain articles written by individuals with specialist knowledge and relevant qualifications in the subject and who will often have conducted the original research as described in the article. Articles are accompanied by extensive citations, a bibliography, and commonly also include an abstract.

Justice: Acting fairly, so that people are treated generally in the same way.

Key informants: Within the context of qualitative research, persons with key, or topic-relevant, information who are interviewed about a particular organization, social program, or problem. They serve as a proxy for their associates within an organization or group. Key informant interviews are in-depth interviews of a select (non-random) group of experts who are most knowledgeable of the organization or issue.

Keyword: A word (or phrase) used when searching an index such as an online database that aids in retrieval of documents. Unlike subject headings, keywords are not part of the subject vocabulary of the database. In full-text searching, every word in a document becomes a keyword. A thesaurus is often constructed to list acceptable keywords.

Keyword searching: The default search in most databases. This option allows the user to enter a significant word or phrase without limiting to any particular field. The results are all records where the search term appears whether in title, author, abstract, notes, subject headings, descriptors, etc., depending on the database. In a library catalogue, the "all fields" word search is equivalent.

Knowledge: The capacity for effective action that results from information, including familiarity, awareness, and understanding gained through experience or study. It results from making comparisons, identifying consequences, and making connections.

Knowledge application: Results in putting knowledge into action in practice settings or circumstances, including adoption, uptake, use, and mobilization. Other terms commonly used for this activity are *adoption*, *uptake*, *utilization*, and *mobilization*. It is also important to figure out how to use evidence appropriately and effectively within the local context (for example, developing a protocol to support a new program is an application activity).

Knowledge broker: An individual or organization that aims to develop relationships and networks with, among, and between producers and users of research evidence and knowledge in order to facilitate: (a) knowledge exchange and co-development, (b) the appropriate use of the best available evidence in decision-making processes, and (c) individual and organizational capacity to participate effectively in the evidence-informed decision-making process.

Knowledge dissemination: The process of pushing out or distributing information, including research evidence, and adapting the content and the means for delivery to be appropriate for the intended audience(s). Activities and tools include briefing documents, educational sessions or workshops, online reviews, summary statements, and publications.

Knowledge exchange: A systematic approach to capture, collect, and share tacit knowledge in order for it to become explicit knowledge. By doing so, this process allows for individuals and organizations to access and utilize essential information, which previously was known intrinsically to only one or a small group of people.

Knowledge management: The systematic application of policies, methods, and tools to create, capture, share, and leverage the knowledge needed for an organization to succeed.

Knowledge mobilization: Collaborative problem-solving between researchers and decision makers that happens through linkage and exchange. Effective knowledge mobilization involves interaction between decision makers and researchers and results in mutual learning through the process of planning, producing, disseminating, and applying existing or new research in decision making.

Knowledge synthesis: A process of assessing current research evidence and expert opinion and providing a more comprehensive perspective on a specific topic.

Syntheses identify gaps in evidence to help establish future research priorities and provide information to support policy and program decision making. The components are identifying a question/problem of interest; establishing criteria to inform study selection; searching literature for relevant research; appraising studies critically; combining study results statistically and thematically; and summarizing synthesis findings.

Knowledge translation: A systematic process for sharing knowledge between researchers and research users, including the synthesis, dissemination, exchange, and ethically sound application of knowledge.

Library collection: The total accumulation of books and other materials owned by a library, catalogued and arranged for ease of access, which often consists of several smaller collections (reference, circulating books, serials, government documents, rare books, special collections, etc.). The process of building a library collection over time is called *collection development*. (Synonymous with holdings.)

Literature review: A literature review is an essay, or introductory matter in a thesis or dissertation, that provides an overview and analysis of the development of a field of study through the published books, articles, essays, and commentary associated with it. Literature reviews can be done in a variety of ways: chronological, thematic, by publication, etc.

Longitudinal: Follow-up over an extended period of time.

Mean: Also called the *average*; the sum of all the observations in a data set divided by the number of observations.

Measurement bias: Bias that occurs when something is measured incorrectly or in an inconsistent manner.

Measurement model: An outcome measures scale and sub-scale structure, which includes direction regarding the procedures to be followed to calculate the scores. This applies to complex instruments that consist of several sub-scales.

Median: The middle value of an ordered set of observations.

Meta-analysis: A systematic review that uses statistical techniques for combining the findings of quantitative studies to produce a summary on a given topic.

Meta-synthesis: An approach to compare and integrate findings from qualitative studies on a given topic.

Methodologies: The broad approaches to research that provide the general framework of the study.

Methods: In the sense they are used in this textbook, the specific tools used to collect data during the research process (e.g., a questionnaire).

Mixed-methods research: A combination of both quantitative and qualitative components, simultaneously or sequentially in the same research project.

Mode: The most frequently occurring number in a data set.

Mortality rate: The death rate in a given population.

Multiple regression: A statistical test to determine the impact of two or more predictor variables (independent) on an outcome variable (dependent).

Multivariate analysis of variance (MANOVA): A statistical test of the differences between the mean scores of two or more groups on two or more outcome variables considered at the same time.

Narrative research: A qualitative design that examines an oral or written story describing a series of events that took place over time.

Narrower term: In a hierarchical classification system, a subject heading or descriptor representing a subclass indicated by another term (for example, "educational psychologist" under "psychologist"). A subject heading or descriptor may have more than one narrower term (also "comparative psychologist" under "psychologist").

Naturalistic: Observation where the activities of one or more individuals are observed where they normally occur, for research purposes.

Non-maleficence: The ethical principle of avoiding doing harm, perhaps better thought of as "first do no harm."

Non-propositional knowledge: See *tacit knowledge*.

Non-profit: An organization that is established for purposes other than directly creating revenue for profit. Information from non-profits can be reliable and accurate. However, **note that some marketing organizations** are created as non-profits to give the appearance of greater credibility and objectivity.

Null hypothesis: A term whereby a hypothesis is posed as the opposite of what the researchers actually expect to find. Null hypotheses are posed for statistical reasons.

Number needed to treat (NNT): The number of patients who need to receive a therapy before one person would experience a beneficial outcome.

Observational studies: Studies that involve observation, which in quantitative research is usually quite structured and in qualitative research much less so. Observational studies do not involve an intervention on the part of the researcher.

Odds ratio (OR): A ratio of the odds (likelihood) of an outcome in one group compared with the odds of the outcome in another group.

Open-ended question: A question that does not appear to suggest an answer, allowing the respondent to give any kind of response.

Operationalize: The process of clearly defining variables in order to establish factors for change or measurement. The process enables some structure and rules to define concepts that may be blurry, relative, or not easily measured (for example, television viewing or coffee drinking) and allows them to be measured, empirically and quantitatively.

Outcome variable (outcome): The characteristic that is measured to find the results. It is also called the *dependent variable*.

Paradigm: The philosophical position that is taken within the research, or the worldview on which the research is based.

Paraphrasing: To restate, concisely and in your own words, the sense or meaning of a text or passage from a book or journal article, etc.

Participant observation: Observing the functioning of a group from within the group.

Participation bias: Influences affecting the sample that participated in the study.

Participatory action research: Research in which the researcher and participating group share ownership of a project to investigate a social problem that involves them, with the intent to empower people and solve problems.

Peer-reviewed research: In academic publishing, a "quality control" and editorial procedure whereby a panel of experts checks (reviews) the validity and accuracy of the content of a document prior to its publication. The peer-review process is a distinguishing feature of scholarly journals and is crucial to maintaining high standards, accuracy, and authority.

Performance bias: Influences affecting care provided or received by either patients or staff because they know that they are in a study. It can sometimes be controlled by placebos.

Periodical index: A collection of citations to journals or magazines. A good periodical index provides numerous access points, from author and title, to subject and publisher, to allow the user to find the needed information.

Phenomenology research: Qualitative research, rooted in philosophy and psychology, that describes or interprets the lived experience of people.

PICO model: Format used to turn a clinical or practical question into a workable search structure by breaking down the question into search terms. The appropriateness of the PICO format will depend on the specific research question and on the type of studies that are suitable for addressing the review question. See also *SPICE*.

> Example Question: *How well does a random urine protein to creatinine ratio diagnose proteinuria versus a 24-hour urine collection for protein?*
>
> **P (population):** The demography of the population (age, gender, race) or the problem of the population (condition or diagnosis or symptoms) (*e.g., people with diabetes*)
>
> **I (intervention):** The treatment under investigation (*e.g., random urine protein to creatinine ratio*)

C (comparator): Comparison of intervention (specific: weight-bearing exercise), alternative interventions (broad: any other treatment), control (nothing) (*e.g., 24-hour urine collection for protein*)

O (outcome): Change in symptoms of the population; reason for using the exposure (*e.g., diagnosis of proteinuria*)

Placebo: An inactive form of a treatment used as a comparison in experiments involving new treatments or interventions.

Placebo effect: A potentially noticeable improvement in someone's condition that is not due to any active intervention. The improvement is, in fact, the result of what is probably a psychological response to attention given to the condition.

Power: The ability of a study to detect statistically significant results using mathematical formulae, depending on the potential sample size as well as the type and frequency of the outcome to be examined.

Pre-post study: Research where one group of subjects is given the same intervention, and this group of subjects acts as its own controls. Outcome measures are taken before (pre, baseline) the intervention is delivered, and the outcome measures are taken again (post-intervention).

Prevalence (prevalent): The amount of a disease in a defined population at a given point in time. If a disease lasts for life, its prevalence will continue to rise, even if the incident rate is low, whereas for a short-lived illness such as a cold or measles, the incidence rate and prevalence will be broadly similar. Often people use the two terms interchangeably, but they are not synonymous.

Primary research: Research conducted and data analyzed directly by a researcher.

Primary research article (paper): A peer-reviewed report of new research on a specific question (or questions).

Primary sources: In scholarship, a document or record containing firsthand information or original data on a topic, used in preparing a derivative work. Primary sources include original manuscripts, periodical articles reporting original research or thought, diaries, memoirs, letters, journals, photographs, drawings, posters, film footage, sheet music, songs, interviews, government documents, public records, eyewitness accounts, and newspaper clippings.

Probability sampling: Sampling that gives everyone in a study population the same chance of being selected for a study as long as they meet the inclusion criteria. When large enough, such sampling produces results that are generalizable to the population from which the sample is drawn.

Propositional knowledge: See *explicit knowledge.*

Prospective: Going forward over time.

Purposive: Refers to a method of sampling within qualitative research whereby people are chosen for inclusion because they meet the purpose of the study. This means they have experience of the phenomenon under study.

p-value: The probability that the result could have occurred by chance if, in reality, the null hypothesis was true. If a result is statistically significant it will be indicated by a p-value. In the case of the value, a scale is assigned to that rating of probability that something will occur, ranging from zero to one.

Qualitative paradigm: A philosophical perspective that frames research interested in discovering truths about how people experience the world and why.

Qualitative research: An inductive, in-depth investigation of phenomena in a holistic fashion that uses a research design concerned with understanding from the qualitative paradigm.

Quality improvement: A method of evaluating and improving the processes of health care, often using a multidisciplinary approach to problem solving.

Quantitative paradigm: A philosophical perspective and position that views the world in a more conventionally scientific sense. People using this paradigm are interested in proving associations, correlations, and cause and effect.

Quantitative research: The investigation of phenomena that uses precise measurement to yield data that are subjected to statistical analysis to respond to questions framed by the quantitative paradigm.

Quasi-experimental studies: Research concerned with comparing measurements and that are usually applied to the observation and measurement of changes that occur naturally (sometimes called *natural experiments*), so it is difficult to control for threats to internal validity. In these studies, the treatment and control groups may not be comparable at baseline or before the intervention/manipulation of the independent variable.

Randomization: The assignment of participants to study groups based on chance (e.g., using a random numbers table). Each participant has an equal probability of being in each study group.

Randomized controlled trial (RCT): A specific form of experiment that is used in the clinical setting in order to compare the usefulness of two or more interventions.

Range: The difference between the largest observation of a data set and the smallest observation.

Realist review: A strategy for synthesizing research that has an explanatory rather than judgmental focus, it seeks to unpack the mechanism of how complex programs work (or why they fail) in particular contexts and settings.

Reasonable expectations of privacy: A term concerned with research ethics. If individuals have reason to expect that information about themselves will normally only be accessed by people within a select group (e.g., family, friends, co-workers, members of an online support group), then they may have a reasonable expectation of privacy.

Recall bias: Bias that occurs when individuals in a study have to rely on their memory in order to answer certain questions. Such biases are created when people who are ill, or have another reason to remember an exposure, are better at recalling events than people who are not ill.

Refereed: See *peer-reviewed research*.

Reference: A conventional word or phrase used in a work to refer the reader to another part of the text ("see above" or "see below") or a similar word or phrase used in an index, catalogue, or reference work to direct the user from one heading or entry to another ("see" or "see also"). It also refers to any Latin phrase used in footnotes, endnotes, and bibliographies to refer the reader to works previously quoted or cited (for example, *ibid.* and *op. cit.*) It is sometimes used synonymously with *citation*. In addition, it can refer to a letter written in support of a person's application for employment or housing, usually by someone familiar with the applicant's qualifications or reputation, or to a person who agrees to be contacted for such a recommendation.

Referencing style: A set of rules for the consistent method of formatting in-text references and bibliographies. The style used may be determined by the subject area, your lecturer, or school (e.g., APA, Harvard, Chicago, MLA, or Vancouver).

Regression analysis: A statistical test to predict an outcome based on the values of one or more factors.

Related terms: A term concerned with searching the literature. It is a descriptor or subject heading closely related to another term conceptually but not hierarchically (for example, "physical therapists" listed as a related term under "health centres").

Relative risk: See *risk ratio.*

Reliability (reliable): It is the consistency with which an instrument measures what it is designed to measure, or the extent to which random variation influences the result. It refers to whether a method of data collection, or measurement, will repeatedly give the same results if used by the same person more than once or by two or more people when measuring the same phenomenon. Reliability can be assessed by testing for (a) stability, i.e., how stable it is over time (test-retest); (b) equivalence, i.e., consistency of the results by different raters (inter-rater reliability) or similar tests at the same time; and (c) internal consistency, i.e., the measurement of the concept is consistent in all parts of the test.

Reporting bias: Influences affecting what results are selected for publication by the researchers or journal editors, such as an increased enthusiasm to publish positive results.

Research: A systematic process used to conduct an investigation in order to generate results that will add to existing evidence.

Research ethics board (REB): A group that reviews the ethical considerations of a research proposal to certify the acceptability of the proposal considering approved ethical standards. They are generally found at a health care institution or university or other large institution.

Research literacy: A term used in health and community practice to describe a set of competencies and abilities to find, understand, critically appraise, and apply research evidence for practice.

Research mindedness: An approach to practice and way of thinking that addresses the significance and relationship of research to practice; awareness, critique, and appreciation of research principles and strategies; and consideration of research in daily life and practice.

Research proposal: A protocol outlining why and how a study will be carried out if permissions are obtained.

Research report: A description of a study that includes why and how it was done, with emphasis on the results.

Research strategy: A plan or scheme by which the activity of searching for and assessing information found is carried out. A search strategy usually involves a number of steps: (a) analyzing the major concepts of the topic; (b) defining relevant keywords and their synonyms; (c) searching appropriate information sources (e.g., databases); and (d) assessing the quantity and quality (relevance) of the information found.

Research utilization: A process by which specific research-based knowledge (science) is implemented in practice.

Response bias: Bias that occurs when individuals respond to a question within a study in a particular way because they think that the answer they are giving is what the researcher wants to hear.

Responsiveness: The degree to which an outcome measure can detect change, often defined as the minimal change considered to be important by a person. Evidence for responsiveness is an important factor when assessing construct validity.

Retrospective: Looking in the past at variables or events that have already occurred.

Review article: Review articles are typically peer-reviewed, but don't present new research information; rather they summarize multiple primary research articles to give a sense of the consensus, debates, and unanswered questions within a field.

Rigour (rigorous): A term used in qualitative research that suggests that the research process has been undertaken in a well-thought-through, well-explained, and transparent manner.

Risk: A statistical term that refers simply to the probability (usually statistical probability) that an event will occur, whether it be a good or a bad event.

Risk ratio (RR): The ratio of risks in an intervention group compared to that of the control group; also called *relative risk* or *weighed mean difference.*

Sample size: The number of participants from a population (whole group) who are selected to participate in a study.

Sampling bias: Bias that occurs when the selection of a sample for a study may exclude certain groups of people in a systematic manner; for example, an online survey will exclude all those people who do not have Internet access.

Scientific method: A systematic approach for investigating phenomena, acquiring new knowledge, or correcting and integrating previous knowledge.

Search engine: A website comprised of a large database of websites. A search engine's spider collects the webpages. The search engine then allows visitors to do keyword searching to find appropriate pages.

Search terms: Keywords or phrases used in a search strategy to retrieve relevant records from a catalogue or library database.

Secondary research: Research carried out by someone else who has data that is then looked at or analyzed again.

Secondary sources: Any published or unpublished work that is one step removed from the original source. Secondary sources usually describe, summarize, analyze, evaluate, derive from, or are based on primary source material (for example, a review, critical analysis, second-hand account, or biographical or historical study). This also refers to material other than primary sources used in the preparation of a written work.

Selection bias: Bias resulting from an action occurring on one side of a study and not the other. For example, if researchers were allowed to decide which participants had which intervention in a study, it is possible that they might select patients they thought would do better in the study or try harder to follow a regime.

Semi-structured interview: A flexible interview in which there is no specific list of questions, only a framework or something like a topic guide for the topics to be addressed.

Sensitivity: How good a test is at detecting who *has* a condition or disease.

Sham treatment (intervention): A fake (placebo) treatment used as a comparison for a new treatment in an experiment such as a randomized controlled trial.

Skepticism: A critical attitude and approach to knowledge.

Specificity: How good a test is at telling who *does not have* the condition or disease.

SPICE model: Format used to turn a clinical question into a workable search structure by breaking down the question into search terms. The appropriateness of the SPICE format will depend on the specific research question and on the type of studies that are suitable for addressing the review question. See also *PICO*.

> Example Question: *What is the impact of an increase in the level of cost-sharing on access to health services for the chronically ill in European countries?*
>
> **S (setting):** What is the context of the question? (*e.g., European countries*)
>
> **P (perspective):** Who are the users/potential users of the outcomes? (*e.g., chronically ill*)
>
> **I (intervention):** What is being done to them? (*e.g., increased cost-sharing*)
>
> **C (comparison):** What are the alternatives? (*e.g., no increase*)
>
> **E (evaluation):** How will you measure if the intervention is successful? (*e.g., access to health services*)

Stakeholder: An individual, group, or organization with a vested interest in the decision to implement a best practice guideline. Stakeholders include all those individuals or groups who will be directly or indirectly affected by, or who can directly or indirectly affect, the implementation of a best practice guideline.

Stakeholder analysis: A stakeholder analysis is the process of identifying and generating information about stakeholders for the purpose of helping the guideline implementation team understand stakeholder behaviour, plans, relationships, and interests. This knowledge can help the team to determine the support, resources, and influences that the stakeholder can bring to bear and determine how best to engage them for success.

Standard deviation: A quantification of the amount of variation of a set of data or values. It is measured by the square root of the variance. The standard deviation enables the researcher and reader to get a feel for where most of the variables within a data set lie.

Statistically significant: The result of a statistical calculation showing a relationship between the variables that is unlikely due to chance alone.

Structuralist theory: A philosophical approach concerned with how individuals behave within a group.

Subjective: A word used to demonstrate that people see the world in different ways, from their own personal perspective.

Survey: Non-experimental research using questionnaires or interviews to obtain information such as beliefs, preferences, attitudes, or activities of people.

Survey study: An observational study that examines a characteristic (or set of characteristics) and the outcome of interest in participants at one point in time. Sometimes referred to as a *cross-sectional study*.

Symbolic interactionism: The study of micro-scale social interactions.

Synthesis: Synthesis in the context of research literacy means the contextualization and integration of research findings of individual research studies within the larger body of knowledge on the topic. A synthesis must be reproducible and transparent in its methods, using quantitative and/or qualitative methods. It could take the form of a systematic review; follow the methods developed by the Cochrane Collaboration; result from a consensus conference or expert panel; and may synthesize qualitative or quantitative results. Realist syntheses, narrative syntheses, meta-analyses, meta-syntheses, and practice guidelines are all forms of synthesis.

Synthesizing: A skill used to analyze and integrate information and develop knowledge of concepts and interpretations (e.g., reading several journal articles to identify common theories from different points of view).

Systematic review: A synthesis or integration of research studies.

Tacit (non-propositional) knowledge: Knowledge that is so deeply embedded that people often forget they have it. It is known to people within a group and does not need explanation within the context of that group, but may be unknown to outsiders.

Temporal effect: An effect that makes sense over a period of time, such as an increase in fatigue over the course of a workday.

Test–retest reliability: Determination of the similarity of results when the same data collection tool is used at different times (e.g., one week apart) with other factors as stable or the consistency of test scores over time based on a correlation between test and retest scores within the same sample. It is assumed that the outcome of interest remains the same over that time period.

Theoretical sampling: A method of sampling that occurs as researchers build new theories and ideas from the data they have collected and test these theories by interviewing more subjects to see if the new theories still hold true. It is usually only a feature of grounded theory research. (Also called *handy sampling*.)

Theory: An understanding about an issue that has been derived by collecting evidence.

Thick description: A detailed account of cultural practices, used in ethnography to present results and provide evidence of rigour.

Timeliness: The quality of being current or timely. The importance of timeliness of sources of information varies depending on its use. For topics relating to current technologies, it is important the information is up-to-date. For other information needs, it may be more relevant to use original or older sources for their historical significance.

Time series design: A research design where data are collected and analyzed over multiple different points in time, typically before and after an intervention.

Tools: For the purposes of this textbook, the term serves to describe standardized products such as instruments, surveys, and checklists that facilitate access to and use of information for knowledge translation and decision making (e.g., a checklist for a dissemination plan).

Topic guides: In interview methods, topic guides are short lists of questions to be used as a way of keeping the interviewer focused on the purpose in an unstructured interview, while allowing some flexibility.

Transferability: A component of qualitative validity, transferability refers to the degree to which the results of qualitative research can be generalized or transferred to other contexts or settings.

Transformative theory: An overarching worldview and approach to study with the intent to empower the participants.

Triangulation: Using multiple sources (methods, data collection, theories) to help validate information.

Trustworthiness: Refers to the rigour (quality) associated with the qualitative research process and results.

t-test: A statistical test used to analyze the difference between two mean scores.

Uncertainty principle: The starting point for all research—because we are uncertain about the answer to a specific question, we undertake research in order to try to remove the uncertainty.

Unstructured interview: An interview that is conducted with few if any guiding questions. These interviews are usually very exploratory in nature.

Validity: The degree to which a data collection tool accurately measures what it is intended to measure. For example, we know that a thermometer (if placed correctly for long enough) will measure temperature, but it is not easy to be certain that a questionnaire designed to measure quality of life actually does so because of the difficulty of defining what "quality of life" actually is. Evidence for the validity of an outcome measure is assessed in three primary ways: criterion, construct, and content validity. See *criterion validity, construct validity,* and *content validity.*

Variable: An attribute or characteristic of a person or object that varies (takes on different values that can be measured in quantitative research, e.g., weight, age, neighbourhood).

Variance: A statistical measure of dispersion (variation) of scores.

Verbatim: Word for word, literally "as something was said."

Vulnerability: Vulnerability is a term used in research ethics. It can be caused by limited capacity, or limited access to social goods, such as rights, opportunities, and power. Anyone can find themselves in vulnerable circumstances at some point in life.

APPENDIX A

PRACTICE EXAM QUESTIONS

1. A basic value of scientific research is
   a) subjectivity
   b) relativity
   c) skepticism
   d) specificity

2. In contrast to science, common or folk knowledge
   a) is guided by our observations
   b) leads us to question our common sense understanding
   c) shapes rather than is shaped by our observations
   d) all of the above

3. Research gathered through the most convenient and accessible information, often in a haphazard way, to solve a particular problem is known as
   a) empirical research
   b) casual research
   c) scientific research
   d) field research

4. What is primary research?
   a) research into a generalizable field of study
   b) research into one very specific topic
   c) research that is at the very origins of the investigation into a topic
   d) research that is carried out by oneself

5. What is secondary research?
    a) the second phase in a multi-phased study of a topic
    b) research somebody else has carried out and that is reported on
    c) research conducted for the purpose of another more in-depth study
    d) research done by oneself

6. Researchers often use _____ to check and reinterpret the findings of other scientists.
    a) primary data analysis
    b) secondary data analysis
    c) national surveys
    d) government documents

7. When using existing data, it is essential to
    a) get permission from the original researchers
    b) have the same theories as the original researchers
    c) understand the aim and purpose of the original research
    d) agree with the original researchers

8. The basic problem with the Internet as a source of factual information is
    a) the sheer volume of material that has to be checked
    b) how easy it is to become distracted by irrelevant information
    c) the small number of reliable sites that can be accessed easily
    d) none of the above

9. Reasoning from specific factual information toward theoretical conclusions is called
    a) inductive logic
    b) deductive logic
    c) analytic logic
    d) common sense

10. Reasoning from theoretical ideas to specific examples is called
    a) abstract logic
    b) inductive logic
    c) deductive logic
    d) systematic logic

11. Setting up a system for the measurement or identification of a change under study is known as
    a) induction
    b) explanation
    c) operationalization
    d) all of the above

12. For the purpose of research, an independent variable is assumed to be the
    a) cause
    b) effect
    c) explanation
    d) measure

13. For the purpose of research, the dependent variable is assumed to be the
    a) measure
    b) cause
    c) effect
    d) explanation

14. Application and utilization of research evidence can be experienced at which areas of practice?
    a) perceived and received paradigms
    b) conceptual and practical levels
    c) pre-contemplative and contemplative phases
    d) relational and collaborative approaches

15. Which of the following is the most common rationale for the lack of research uptake?
    a) the ethical dilemmas found in research methods
    b) the professional and patient perspectives on the change
    c) the realities of timing and resources (human, material, and skills resources)
    d) the challenges of interpretation of findings

16. Disseminating research aims to accomplish which tasks in the research process?
    a) interpreting findings
    b) evaluating the quality of research
    c) analyzing data
    d) contributing to the searchable evidence base

17. Knowledge mobilization activities aim to support research and practice by
    a) accelerating the use of evidence in practice
    b) applying culturally sensitive terms to findings
    c) interpreting research findings with more accuracy
    d) generating knowledge faster

18. Which of the following explains the research-to-practice gap?
    a) few applied forums to disseminate research to practitioners
    b) resistance to change
    c) volume and pace of information produced
    d) all of the above

Practice Exam Answers
  1. Ans: C
  2. Ans: C
  3. Ans: B
  4. Ans: D
  5. Ans: B
  6. Ans: B
  7. Ans: C
  8. Ans: A
  9. Ans: A
10. Ans: C
11. Ans: C
12. Ans: A
13. Ans: C
14. Ans: B
15. Ans: C
16. Ans: D
17. Ans: A
18. Ans: D

APPENDIX B

LEARNING ACTIVITIES

CHAPTER 1 LEARNING ACTIVITY

Activity 1.1: Why Is Research Important for Evidence-Informed Practice?

1. Read the following scenario and reflect on how you would proceed and how research would contribute:

   Assume that you are the program director of a community health centre. A child wellness advocacy group comes to you wanting to know the best ways to address the current childhood obesity problem identified by families, schools, and community programs.

2. By yourself or in a pair, write down an everyday problem in your community or health practice (or your everyday work or life outside of these professional fields); for instance, a problem of choosing one approach over another, difficulty with scheduling and implementing an activity, or an issue of the environment and the context of a problem.

3. List some of the ways that research may help in decision making or acting on the problem you have identified.

CHAPTER 2 LEARNING ACTIVITIES

Activity 2.1: Types of Knowledge: Identifying Information, Research, and Knowledge in the News

1. Work with one or two other learners.
2. Find an online news source. Go through listings to find the following:
    *   **One** article that describes research findings of some sort
    *   **One** article that refers to numbers, but you don't think it is research
3. Determine what the similarities and differences are between the two articles. Look for at least two similarities and two differences. Consider the following:
    *   Whom is the article written for?
    *   Who is doing the writing?
    *   Why would someone think these discoveries were important enough to publish as news?
4. Describe the kind of knowledge each article is providing (tacit, explicit, practical, speculative).
5. Fill out the following table.

Table A.1: Knowledge in the News

	Article One	Article Two
What is this article about?		
Similarities (at least two)		
Differences (at least two)		

(continued)

Table A.1: Knowledge in the News (continued)

Kind of knowledge the article provides (tacit, explicit, practical, speculative, etc.). Give rationale for your choice.		
What other questions does this information lead you to ask? What other research questions might be asked to follow up these discoveries posted in the news?		

Activity 2.2: Issues, Problem, Sub-problem, and Research Question Explorations

Researchable problems range from simple to complex, depending on the context, number of variables, and the nature of their relationship. If you understand the nature of the *problem*, you will be able to better understand where to look for research that can inform your practice.

1. Identify an issue in professional practice (or even an everyday life concern).
2. Create a mind-map, listing the environment and context of the problem with associated problems and related sub-problems.
3. Review the list of the initial practice (or everyday life) issue, contextual issues, and sub-problems. Identify priority research questions to be explored.

CHAPTER 3 LEARNING ACTIVITY

Activity 3.1: Disciplinary, Philosophical, and Theoretical Influences

Influenced by different philosopies and theories, researchers from different disciplines and professional practice fields have varying approaches to their problems in health and community practice.

1. List the professional practice disciplines that would be interested in exploring the listed issues.
2. Consider what questions might be asked of the following research problems from inductive and deductive research paradigms.

Table A.2

Practice Problem/Issue	Interested Professional Practice Disciplines	Question Underpinned by Inductive (Qualitative) Paradigm	Question Underpinned by Deductive (Quantitative) Paradigm
Your client who is homeless is malnourished.			
Your patient has a laceration on his left eye from a domestic dispute.			
Your client is anxious about genetic testing for her first pregnancy.			

CHAPTER 4 LEARNING ACTIVITIES

Activity 4.1: Search and Identify Research Relevance and Credibility

This learning activity is designed to give you practical experience in searching for and identifying a research study in a topic of your interest.

1. Search for a research paper in a topic of your interest.
2. Review the article with a view to identifying the *relevance* to your questions/interests:
   - Identify the **purpose** of each study.
   - Identify **what is being "done"** in each study.
   - Identify the **research methodology** used.
   - Identify the **sample size**.
   - Identify the **main result**.
3. Identify the general credibility of the research paper:
   - Check to see if there is a match between the **research topic** and the **qualifications** of the authors (education, practice designation, and the institutions within which they practice).
   - Check the type and **reputation of the information source** (e.g., academic versus trade journal or magazine, impact factor, peer-reviewed versus not peer-reviewed).
   - Check for **signs of "scholarliness"** (e.g., the article has the expected sections of a research article if it is a research article; the authors have been careful with spelling, punctuation, and grammar; there is a substantial reference list; the article has been assigned a "doi"; the keywords are consistent with the professional vocabulary of the relevant discipline and match the thesauruses of the databases used for the literature review to ensure a comprehensive search).
   - Check to see if the **significance** (meaningfulness and importance) of the research question is well supported in the introduction section of the research report.
   - Check for evidence that the research or information gathering has been done in an **ethical** manner (e.g., check for ethics board approval).

Activity 4.2: Identifying Research Integrity in the Literature Review

A good literature review highlights different perspectives and trends and presents an argument about what is already known in the literature on a certain topic. In doing so, the literature review identifies research gaps and questions to be explored in a new research study. Reading for these arguments is crucial to understanding the purpose and underlying direction of research.

1. Find two research papers in a topic of your interest and carefully read the literature these authors review. List the two citations.
2. For each citation, list the key perspectives and trends the authors identify in the literature. Describe the main arguments the authors make for conducting their research studies in response to the existing literature.
3. Appraise the strengths and weaknesses of the literature review in each research paper.

CHAPTER 5 LEARNING ACTIVITY

Activity 5.1: Appraisal of Research Integrity—Ethical Aspects of Research

Below are six vignettes that describe different research scenarios that involve possibly questionable ethical decisions.

1. Place each situation in one of the following groups: no violation, minor violation, moderate violation, or severe violation.
2. Rank order these situations in terms of how seriously they violate the principles of ethical research on humans.
3. Explain the reasons for your rankings.
4. For each of the situations, identify what you believe to be the one or two ethical principles that are most apparent in that situation. Explain why.

Vignettes:
a) In an introductory class, a sociology instructor asks students to complete questionnaires that the instructor will analyze and use in preparing a journal article for publication.
b) After a field study of deviant behaviour during a riot, law enforcement officials demand that a researcher identify those persons who were observed looting. Rather than risk arrest as an accomplice after the fact, the researcher complies.
c) A researcher promises participants in a study a summary of the results. Later, due to a budget cut, the summary is not sent out.
d) After completing the final draft of a book reporting a research project, an author discovers that 25 of the 2,000 survey interviews were falsified by interviewers, but chooses to ignore this and publishes the book anyway.
e) A researcher discovers that 85 percent of students smoke marijuana regularly at school. Publication of this finding will probably create a furor in the community. Because no extensive analysis of drug use is planned, the researcher decides to ignore the finding and not mention it in the report.
f) A graduate student joins an Internet discussion board about the sports car she drives. She occasionally posts some responses on the board and decides to do a sociological study about the sense of community experienced by members. She attends a car rally sponsored by the board and mingles with participants. She uses archived discussion posts and notes she kept while at car rallies for her study.

CHAPTER 6 LEARNING ACTIVITIES

Activity 6.1: Appraisal of Research Credibility for a Qualitative Research Paper

1. Search for a qualitative research paper in a health and community practice topic of your choice.
2. List the citation.
3. Provide rationale: List three to four elements of this article that help you identify it as a *qualitative* piece of research (consider the problem/question, methods chosen, data presented, reasoning).
4. Appraise its research credibility: Appraise the type and quality of the journal, the authors' credentials, and the review process. Identify the purpose of the research and how the findings are presented. Describe if and how the authors are convincing in their argument, and if you believe the conclusions reached are appropriate given the findings presented in the article.

Activity 6.2: Appraisal of Research Integrity: Questions to Ask When Reading a Qualitative Research Paper

1. Select a qualitative research paper in a health and community practice area of your interest.
2. Appraise the integrity of the research using the questions in the following table (A3).
3. Write your critique in a narrative summary.

Table A.3

1. Citation	What is the name of the paper? The complete citation?
2. Purpose and study rationale	Did the authors provide a clear statement of the aims of the research?
3. Fit and specific rationale	Is a qualitative methodology appropriate?
4. Design	Was the research design appropriate to address the aims of the research?
5. Participants	Was the recruitment strategy appropriate to the aims of the research?
6. Researcher (or researchers)	Has the relationship between researcher and participants been adequately considered?
7. Ethics	Have ethical issues been taken into consideration?
8. Context	Where did the study take place?
9. Data	What was the sequence of the study? Were the data collected in a way that addressed the research issue?
10. Analysis	Was the analysis of the data sufficiently rigorous?
11. Findings and results	Was there a clear statement of findings?
12. Conclusions	What did the authors assert about how the results and study process contribute to the conclusions?
13. Implications and application	How valuable is the research?

Source: Adapted from "Understanding and Critiquing Qualitative Research Papers," by P. Lee, 2006, *Nursing Times, 102*(29), pp. 30–32. Copyright 2006 by Lee; and *Reading and Understanding Research* (3rd ed.), L.F. Locke, S.J. Silverman & W.W. Spirduso, 2010, London, United Kingdom: Sage. Copyright 2010 by Lee et al.

CHAPTER 7 LEARNING ACTIVITIES

Activity 7.1: Reading and Understanding Integrity Issues in Quantitative Research Design

Work solo or with a partner. Read the following random experiment scenario and answer the following questions.

Random Experiment Scenario: "Harmony Hospice Volunteer Training"
The objective of this experiment was to determine the effect that online training modules and support have on volunteer experiences. A random sample of hospice volunteers who participated in a larger program of training was selected. Subjects were randomly assigned either to a treatment group, who received specific online training modules with individual instructor support in addition to an on-site, group training program of one evening a week over the course of six weeks, or to a control group, who received no online module support and only received the six-week group training.

After completing the training experience, each subject completed a questionnaire. It consisted of 10 questions that evaluated the subject's understanding of the training materials and potential responses to hospice volunteer work scenarios, as well as personal comfort and satisfaction with their volunteer role. They consisted of questions such as "How likely would you be to recommend that someone else volunteer for Harmony Hospice?"; "How comfortable do you feel responding to family members of the dying who are experiencing a range of emotions?"; "How do you rate the time commitment involved in your volunteer training?"; "How do you rate the quality of support available to you during the training?"

All responses ranged from 1 (very negative) to 5 (very positive). The responses for each subject were added to give an overall "appreciation rating": e.g., an individual who responded 3, 4, 2, 3, 4, 3, 2, 1, 2, 3 received a rating of 27.

Harmony Hospice Volunteer Training: Random Experiment Questions

1. In your own words, what was the objective or purpose of this random experiment?
2. List the independent variable(s) received by the treatment group. How were these subjects assigned to this group?
3. Who was in the control group? How were these subjects assigned to this group?
4. Discuss the strengths and weaknesses of this study design. What changes would you make to the design?

Activity 7.2: Appraisal of Research Integrity: Questions to Ask When Reading a Quantitative Research Paper

1. Select a quantitative research paper in a health and community practice area of your interest.
2. Appraise the integrity of the research using the questions in the following table (A4).
3. Write your critique in a narrative summary.

Table A.4

1. Citation	What is the study report? The complete citation?
2. Purpose and study rationale	Did the authors provide a clear statement of the aims of the research?
3. Fit and specific rationale	Is a quantitative methodology appropriate?
4. Design	Was the research design appropriate to address the aims of the research?
5. Participants	Was the recruitment strategy appropriate to the aims of the research? Are the sampling issues relevant to the methodology adequately addressed? Does the sampling strengthen or weaken the quality of the results?
6. Researcher (or researchers)	Has the relationship between researcher and participants been adequately considered?
7. Ethics	Have ethical issues been taken into consideration?
8. Context	Where did the study take place?
9. Data	What was the sequence of the study? What constituted data (e.g., test scores, questionnaire responses, etc.) and were data collected to address validity and reliability concerns?
10. Analysis	What form of data analysis was used, and what specific question was it designed to answer? What statistical operations and computer programs were employed?
11. Findings and results	What are identified as the primary results (products of findings produced by the data analysis)?
12. Conclusions	What did the authors assert about how the results and study process contribute to the conclusions?
13. Implications and application	How valuable is the research? Consider generalizability and any limitations.

Source: Adapted from *Reading and Understanding Research* (3rd ed.), L.F. Locke, S.J. Silverman & W.W. Spirduso, 2010, London, United Kingdom: Sage. Copyright 2010 by Lee et al.

CHAPTER 8 LEARNING ACTIVITY

Activity 8.1: Bringing Evidence to Health and Community Practice: Everyday Research Questions

As a health and community practitioner, you are asked to rapidly synthesize evidence in order to respond to everyday problems and questions. Your literacy and communication of a thoughtful and informed response is important for your professional credibility.

1. In a small group, select a question from the list of everyday research questions provided below.
2. In your small group, consider a response based on "best evidence" for the case scenarios provided—search the evidence, then critically appraise and summarize the decision based on the best evidence.
3. Prepare a short presentation (create a brief PowerPoint or Prezi presentation) for the class, critically citing from the evidence. Prepare to face questions and debate based on your argument!

Everyday Research Questions

Choose from the 17 scenarios below, or create one based on a question you have been asked in your practice or everyday life:

a) At a family reunion your 75-year-old great-aunt tells you she is throwing away her pots and pans, stating, "*I heard all those aluminum pots and pans are bad for mental alertness and cause Alzheimer's.*" Your family disagrees. She asks, "*What have you heard?*" What do you tell her based on the latest evidence?

b) One of your friends is very anxious over the fact that she used marijuana weekly or so while in high school: "*I was just goofing around, experimenting, and sort of in the wrong crowd, but now I want to finish my education and have a great job.*" Her anxiety is heightened because she recently heard on a television show that "marijuana can cause schizophrenia." What can you tell her?

c) One of your classmates has said that he would like to replace his "sitting" desk with a "standing" desk. He's heard that when you stand to study, it decreases back discomfort and burns more calories than sitting. One of his roommates thinks that such claims are not well-substantiated and that this is just a fad. Another roommate, who is a nursing student, says he recently saw something on the news about these "standing" desks, saying that they are ergonomically better for you than the sitting desks. How can you help these two roommates with their differing opinions?

d) Your Mom swears by ginseng, taking the herbal supplement at the slightest hint of any cold. Your Dad thinks it is a scam that is costing them a lot of money. They ask you, "*Who wins this argument anyway?*" What do you have to tell them?

e) Your friends love to party at the university bar (especially on "student night"); they claim that caffeine and energy drinks are the solution to a bit of flagging energy for early morning classes on the mornings after. Does your best evidence support or refute this claim about "energy drinks" and hangovers?

f) Your cousin is getting married in June. She has heard that drinking green tea can speed up her weight loss efforts before the big day and has bought every variety that can be found in a desperate effort. Is she wasting her money or could it help her waistline (and in what dose)?

g) Your Aunt Jane is convinced the magnet therapy bracelet she has bought (at considerable expense) is producing a therapeutic effect for her arthritis pain and functioning. Your cousin is livid that she keeps getting taken advantage of by "quacks" at health fairs and on the Internet. Much to your cousin's dismay, your aunt is considering investing in more magnet therapy products. Help them in the dilemma that is causing considerable family tension! What can you tell your aunt and cousin from the best evidence?

h) Your roommates are in an intense debate over the merits of using antibacterial hand wash as a soap and water alternative. One says she has heard that the drying effect breaks the skin, creating more threats of contamination; the other says, "*How could cleaning be a problem? No matter what, it is better to kill bacteria.*" The debate gets turned over to you since you are almost a nurse. Who wins the battle over hand wash?

i) Your dad likes to have a few drinks after work and keeps saying, "*I heard that red wine is good for your health.*" Others in the family disagree and think he is just looking for an excuse to drink. Are there really health benefits to red wine or is this messaging a bunch of hype?

j) Your older sister has let you know that she is embarrassed to say it, but that she has occasionally spanked her three-year old: "*Gently, and always to stop what is a tantrum that is just swirling out of control.*" She says she never talks about it because there is so much stigma about spanking, and that she is worried people would consider it abusive, even though she is very conscious of not hurting your little nephew. In conversation, she asks you if you think there is any research out there that proves spanking causes violence in children in later life. What can you tell her that you find in your search? What is the recommended best practice for disciplining behaviour that is out of control?

k) Recently, two young adults in your circle of family and friends have been diagnosed with brain tumours. Your stepmother raises her concern of cell phone use, asking you, *"Since you're in university, what do you know about this?"* and asks whether she should allow your younger siblings to use them. What could you say is the best evidence-informed decision?

l) Your old high school friend Steve is an occasional pot smoker, *"just at festivals or social things—maybe once or twice a month."* His wife used to be a bit of a partier too, but doesn't partake anymore. She says she sees how it takes away Steve's motivation, so she wants to see him quit once and for all. Steve says, *"It is better than hangovers"* and *"There is no scientific proof the occasional puff takes away motivation."* Because you are a university student, they ask you what the final word is on the matter of motivation and marijuana.

m) Your roommate is a self-confessed "germ freak," and insists on all manner of antibacterial soaps and products as well as a regular good old bleach wipe-down of the counters, fridge, and bathroom fixtures. You are a more "relaxed" homemaker, and so the arguments are routine at your apartment. You are of the belief that everyone needs to be exposed to a few germs to "build up immunity." Will you have to clean up your act, or can you make your case based on the latest evidence?

n) Is chocolate good for your health—yes or no—and, if so, in what dose? Do the rewards balance out the risks? What does the evidence say?

o) Your sister has been hassling you about your choice to wear makeup—especially that bright red lipstick and nail polish you like to apply most days—with routine touch ups! She claims that the combined effects of all the cosmetics, toxins in other beauty products like shampoos, and so on, along with various other contaminants you are exposed to are carcinogenic. What does the evidence advise?

p) You heard in a support group that "persons of faith" tend to handle recovering from an illness better than persons without a faith. One of your classmates challenges you by saying, *"I've heard that how a person handles recovering from an illness has nothing to do with one's faith, but with a positive attitude."* How can you help this classmate with these differing opinions?

q) Growing up, you didn't eat many eggs because you were told *"Too many eggs are bad for you, as they cause an increase in cholesterol level."* Recently, you've heard that such a claim is unfounded, and that one can eat eggs without any adverse effects on one's health. What's the truth?

CHAPTER 9 LEARNING ACTIVITY

Activity 9.1: Infographics and Job Aids: Drawing Research to Practice

1. Locate a relevant infographic and job aid (at least one of each) for your practice area of interest. List all citations and links.
2. List the best practice recommendations and relevant dissemination for the tools.
3. Appraise the tools considering the **credibility** and **integrity** of the evidence that has informed the instructions and information.
4. Comment on any changes or updates you would recommend.

REFERENCES

ADAPTE Collaboration. (2009). *Guideline adaptation: A resource toolkit* (Version 2). Retrieved from www.g-i-n.net/document-store/working-groups-documents/adaptation/adapte-resource-toolkit-guideline-adaptation-2-0.pdf

Agency for Healthcare Research and Quality. (n.d.). *National guideline clearinghouse.* Retrieved August 11, 2016, from www.guideline.gov

Ajetunmobi, O. (2001). *Making sense of critical appraisal.* London, UK: Arnold.

American Psychological Association. (2010). *Publication manual of the American Psychological Association* (6th ed.). Washington, DC: Author.

Baker, C.M., Ogden, S.J., Prapaipanich, W., Keith, C.K., Beattie, L.C., & Nickleson, L. (1999). Hospital consolidation: Applying stakeholder analysis to merger life cycle. *Journal of Nursing Administration, 29*(3), 11–20.

Beck, C.T. (1993). Qualitative research: The evaluation of its credibility, fittingness, and auditability. *Western Journal of Nursing Research, 15,* 263–266. http://dx.doi.org/10.1177/019394599301500212

Bero, L.A., Grilli, R., Grimshaw, J.M., Harvey, E., Oxman, A.D., & Thomson, M.A. (1998). Closing the gap between research and practice: An overview of systematic reviews of interventions to promote the implementation of research findings. *BMJ: British Medical Journal, 317,* 465–468. http://dx.doi.org/10.1136/bmj.317.7156.465

Bonato, S. (2013). *Googling the Greys: Tips for Searching Beyond Health Databases and Turning Information into Insights.* Retrieved from www.lib.uwaterloo.ca/staff/isrtrain/sessions/documents/googlinggreys.pdf

Booth, A. (2006). Clear and present questions: Formulating questions for evidence based practice. *Library Hi Tech, 24,* 355–368. http://dx.doi.org/10.1108/07378830610692127

Bouma, G.D., Ling, R., & Wilkinson, L. (2012). *The research process* (2nd Canadian ed.). Toronto, Canada: Oxford University Press.

Brigham and Women's Hospital, Harvard Medical School & Harvard T.H. Chan School of Public Health. (2016). *Nurses' health study.* Retrieved August 11, 2016, from www.nurseshealthstudy.org

Brouwers, M., Kho, M.E., Browman, G.P., Burgers, J.S., Cluzeau, F., Feder, G., ... Zitzelsberger, L. (2010). AGREE II: Advancing guideline development, reporting and evaluation in healthcare. *Canadian Medical Association Journal, 182,* e839–e842. http://dx.doi.org/10.1503/cmaj.090449

Burls, A. (2009). *What is critical appraisal?* (2nd ed.). Oxford, UK: University of Oxford.

Burns, N., & Grove, S.K. (2011). *Understanding nursing research* (5th ed.). Toronto, Canada: W.B. Saunders Company.

Canadian Institutes of Health Research, Natural Sciences and Engineering Research Council of Canada, & Social Sciences and Humanities Research Council of Canada (TCPS2). (2014). *Tri-council policy statements: Ethical conduct for research involving humans.* Retrieved from www.pre.ethics.gc.ca/pdf/eng/tcps2-2014/TCPS_2_FINAL_Web.pdf.

Canadian Medical Association. (2016). *CPG infobase.* Retrieved from August 11, 2016, www.cma.ca/En/Pages/clinical-practice-guidelines.aspx

Carnwell, R. (2001). Essential differences between research and evidence-based practice. *Nurse Researcher, 8*(2), 55–68. http://dx.doi.org/10.7748/nr2001.01.8.2.55.c6150

Center for History and New Media. (2016). Zotero [Referencing software] (Version 4). Retrieved from www.zotero.org

Charmaz, K. (2006). *Constructing grounded theory: A practical guide through qualitative analysis.* Thousand Oaks, CA: Sage.

CILIP Information Literacy Group. (2014). *Information Literacy Group.* Retrieved August 11, 2016, from www.cilip.org.uk/about/special-interest-groups/information-literacy-group

Ciliska, D., Thomas, H., & Buffett, C. (2008). *An introduction to evidence-informed public health and a compendium of critical appraisal tools for public health practice.* Hamilton, Canada: National Collaborating Centre for Methods and Tools.

Clandinin, D.J. (2007). *Handbook of narrative inquiry: Mapping a methodology.* Los Angeles, CA: Sage.

Colaizzi, P.F. (1978). Psychological research as the phenomenologist views it. In R.S. Valle & M. King (Eds.), *Existential phenomenological alternatives for psychology* (pp. 48–71). New York: Plenum.

Concato, J. (2004). Observational versus experimental studies: What's the research for a hierarchy? *NeuroRx, 1*, 341–347. http://dx.doi.org/10.1602/neurorx.1.3.341

Cooke, A., Smith, D., & Booth, A. (2012). Beyond PICO: The SPIDER tool for qualitative evidence synthesis. *Qualitative Health Research, 22*, 1435–1443. http://dx.doi .org/10.1177/1049732312452938

Creswell, J. W. (2014). *Research design: Qualitative, quantitative, and mixed methods approaches* (4th ed.). Los Angeles, CA: Sage.

Critical Appraisal Skills Programme. (2013). *Critical appraisal skills programme (CASP).* Retrieved August 11, 2016, from http://www.casp-uk.net

Daly, J., Willis, K., Small, R., Green, J., Welch, N., Kealy, M., & Hughes, E. (2007). A hierarchy of evidence for assessing qualitative health research. *Journal of Clinical Epidemiology, 60*(1), 43–49. http://dx.doi.org/10.1016/j.jclinepi.2006.03.014

Davies, B., Edwards, N., Ploeg, J., & Virani, T. (2008). Insights about the process and impact of implementing nursing guidelines on delivery of care in hospitals and community settings. *BMC Health Services Research, 8*(1), 29. http://dx.doi.org/10.1186/1472-6963-8-29

Davis, D.A., & Taylor-Vaisey, A. (1997). Translating guidelines into practice. A systematic review of theoretic concepts, practical experience and research evidence in the adoption of clinical practice guidelines. *Canadian Medical Association Journal, 157*, 408–416.

Denys, K., Rasmussen, C., & Henneveld, D. (2011). The effectiveness of a community-based intervention for parents with FASD. *Community Mental Health Journal, 47*, 209–219. http://dx.doi.org/10.1007/s10597-009-9273-9

Dey, I. (2007). Grounding Categories. In: Bryant, A., Charmaz, K. (Eds.). *The Sage Handbook of Grounded Theory* (pp.167–190). London, UK: Sage.

DiCenso, A., Bayley, L., & Haynes, R.B. (2009). Accessing pre-appraised evidence: Fine-tuning the 5S model into a 6S model. *Evidence-Based Nursing, 12*, 99–101. http://dx.doi.org/10.1136/ebn.12.4.99-b

Dunifon, R. (2005). *How to read a research article.* Retrieved from www.iith.ac.in/rsportal/wp-content/uploads/2014/09/How-to-Read-a-Research-Article.pdf

Edson, W.N., Koniz-Booher, P., Boucar, M., Djbrina, S., & Mahamane, I. (2002). The role of research in developing job aids for pneumonia treatment in Niger. *International Journal for Quality in Health Care, 14*(Suppl. 1), 35–45. http://dx.doi.org/10.1093/intqhc/14.suppl_1.35

Edwards, I., & Jones, M.A. (2007). Clinical reasoning and expertise. In G.M. Jensen, J. Gwyer, L.M. Hack & K. Shepard (Eds.), *Expertise in physical therapy practice* (2nd ed., pp. 192–213). Boston, MA: Elsevier.

El Hussein, M., Jakubec, S. L., & Osuji, J. (2015). Assessing the FACTS: A mnemonic for teaching and learning the rapid assessment of rigor in qualitative research studies. *The Qualitative Report, 20*, 1182–1184.

Ellis, P. (2013). *Understanding research for nursing students* (2nd ed.). Thousand Oaks, CA: Sage.

Elsevier. (2016). *Scopus.* Retrieved August 11, 2016, from www.scopus.com

Farace, D.J., & Schöpfel, J. (2010). *Grey literature in library and information studies.* New York, NY: De Gruyter Saur.

Ferguson-Paré, M., Closson, T., & Tully, S. (2002). Nursing best practice guidelines: A gift for advancing professional practice in every environment. *Hospital Quarterly, 5*(3), 66–68. http://dx.doi.org/10.12927/hcq.16516

Field, M.J., & Lohr, K.N. (1992). *Guidelines for clinical practice: From development to use.* Washington, DC: National Academy Press.

Finch, P.M. (2007). The evidence funnel: Highlighting the importance of research literacy in the delivery of evidence informed complementary health care. *Journal of Bodywork & Movement Therapies, 11*(1), 78–81. http://dx.doi.org/10.1016/j.jbmt.2006.09.001

Fineout-Overholt, E., & Johnston, L. (2005). Teaching EBP: Asking searchable, answerable clinical questions. *Worldviews on Evidence-Based Nursing, 2*, 157–160. http://dx.doi.org/10.1111/j.1741-6787.2005.00032.x

Fitchett, G., Tartaglia, A., Dodd-McCue, D., & Murphy, P. (2012). Educating chaplains for research literacy: Results of a national survey of clinical pastoral education residency programs. *The Journal of Pastoral Care & Counseling: JPCC, 66*(1), 3–3. doi:10.1177/154230501206600103

Fixen, D., Naoom, S.F., Blase, K.A., Friedman, R.M., & Wallace, F. (2005). *Implementation research: A synthesis of the literature.* Retrieved from http://ctndisseminationlibrary.org/PDF/nirnmonograph.pdf

Gabbay, J., & le May, A. (2004). Evidence-based guidelines or collectively constructed "mindlines"? Ethnographic study of knowledge management in primary care. *BMJ: British Medical Journal, 329*, 1013–1016. http://dx.doi.org/10.1136/bmj.329.7473.1013

Gerstman, B.B. (2015). *Basic biostatistics: Statistics for public health practice.* Burlington, MA: Jones & Bartlett Learning.

Gibbs, L.E. (2003). *Evidence-based practice for the helping professions: A practical guide with integrated multimedia.* Pacific Grove, CA: Brooks/Cole–Thomson Learning.

Gomm, R. (2000a). Should we afford it? In R. Gomm & C. Davies (Eds.), *Using evidence in health and social care* (pp. 192–211). London, UK: Sage.

Gomm, R. (2000b). Would it work here? In R. Gomm & C. Davies (Eds.), *Using evidence in health and social care* (pp. 171–191). London, UK: Sage.

Google. (n.d.). *How search works: From algorithms to answers.* Retrieved from www.google.ca /insidesearch/howsearchworks/thestory/

Gordis, L. (2008). *Epidemiology* (7th ed.). Philadelphia, PA: Saunders.

Graham, I.D., & Harrison, M.B. (2005). Evaluation and adaptation of clinical practice guidelines. *Evidence-Based Nursing, 8*(3), 68–72. http://dx.doi.org/10.1136/ebn.8.3.68

Graham, I.D, Logan, J., Harrison, M.B., Straus, S.E., Tetroe, J., Caswell, W., & Robinson, N. (2006). Lost in knowledge translation: Time for a map? *Journal of Continuing Education in the Health Professions, 26*(1):13–24. doi: 10.1002/chp.47.

Greenhalgh, T. (2006). *How to read a paper: The basics of evidence-based medicine* (3rd ed.). London, UK: BMJ.

Greenhalgh, T. (2014). *How to read a paper: The basics of evidence-based practice* (5th ed.). Hoboken, NJ: Wiley-Blackwell.

Guba, E.G., & Lincoln, Y.S. (1989). *Fourth generation evaluation.* Newbury Park, CA: Sage.

Guba, E.G., & Lincoln, Y.S. (1994). Competing paradigms in qualitative research. In N.K. Denzin & Y.S. Lincoln (Eds.), *Handbook of qualitative research* (pp. 105–117). London, UK: Sage.

Guyatt, G.H., Sackett, D.L., Sinclair, J.C., Hayward, R., Cook, D.J., & Cook, R.J. (1995). Users' guides to the medical literature. IX. A method for grading health care recommendations. Evidence-Based Medicine Working Group. *Journal of the American Medical Association, 274,* 1800–1804. http://dx.doi.org/10.1001/jama.1995.03530220066035

Hamajima, N., Hirose, K., Tajima, K., Rohan, T., Calle, E.E., Heath Jr., C.W., et al. (2002). Collaborative group on hormonal factors in breast cancer. Alcohol, tobacco and breast cancer— collaborative reanalysis of individual data from 53 epidemiological studies, including 58,515 women with breast cancer and 95,067 women without the disease. *British Journal of Cancer, 87,* 1234-1245. http://dx.doi.org/10.1038/sj.bjc.6600596

Harrison, M.B., Graham, I.D., & Fervers, B. (2009). Adapting knowledge to a local context. In S. Straus, J. Tetroe & I. Graham (Eds.), *Knowledge translation in health care: Moving from evidence to practice* (pp. 73–82). London, UK: Wiley.

Hayden, E.C. (2013). Geneticists push for global data-sharing. *Nature, 498*(7452):16–7. doi:10.1038/498017a.

Health Canada. (2006). *Best practices: Early intervention, outreach and community linkages for women with substance use problems.* Retrieved from www.hc-sc.gc.ca/hc-ps/alt_formats/hecs-sesc/pdf /pubs/adp-apd/early-intervention-precoce/early-intervention-precoce-eng.pdf

Health Evidence™. (2013). *Developing an efficient strategy using P.S.* Retrieved from www.healthevidence. org/documents/practice-tools/HETools_DevelopingEfficientSearchStrategyUsingPICO_18. Mar.2013.doc

Hearns, G., Klein, M.C., Trousdale, W., Ulrich, C., Butcher, D., Miewald, C., ... Procyk, A. (2010). Development of a support tool for complex decision-making in the provision of rural maternity care. *Healthcare Policy, 5*(3), 82–96. http://dx.doi.org/10.12927/hcpol.2013.21641

Herttua, K., Mäkelä, P., Martikainen, P., & Sirén, R. (2008). The impact of a large reduction in the price of alcohol on area differences in interpersonal violence: A natural experiment based on aggregate data. *Journal of Epidemiology & Community Health, 62*, 99–1001. http://dx.doi.org/10.1136/jech.2007.069575

Higgs, J., Fish, D., & Rothwell, R. (2008). Knowledge generation and clinical reasoning in practice. In J. Higgs, M.A. Jones, S. Loftus, & N. Christensen (Eds.), *Clinical reasoning in the health professions* (3rd ed., pp. 163–172). Philadelphia, PA: Elsevier.

Higgs, J., Jones, M.A., & Titchen, A. (2008). Knowledge, reasoning and evidence for practice. In J. Higgs, M. Jones, S. Loftus, & N. Christensen (Eds.), *Clinical reasoning in the health professions,* (3rd ed., pp. 151–162). Philadelphia, PA: Elsevier.

Higuchi, K.S., Davies, B.L., Edwards, N., Ploeg, J., & Virani, T. (2011). Implementation of clinical guidelines for adults with asthma and diabetes: A three-year follow-up evaluation of nursing care. *Journal of Clinical Nursing, 20*, 1329–1338. http://dx.doi.org/10.1111/j.1365-2702.2010.03590.x

Hines, S., Ramsbotham, J., & Coyer, F. (2015). The effectiveness of interventions for improving the research literacy of nurses: A systematic review. *Worldviews on Evidence-Based Nursing, 12*, 265–272. http://dx.doi.org/10.1111/wvn.12106

How to read a paper: Papers that summarise other papers (systematic reviews and meta-analyses). (1997). *BMJ, 315,* 672. http://dx.doi.org/10.1136/bmj.315.7109.672

Institute of Medicine. (2011). *Clinical practice guidelines we can trust.* Retrieved from www.iom.edu/Reports/2011/Clinical-Practice-Guidelines-We-Can-Trust.asp

Jakubec, S.L. (2015). Research literacy. In M.J. Smith, R. Carpenter, & J.J. Fitzpatrick (Eds.), *Encyclopedia of nursing education* (pp. 297–299). New York, NY: Springer.

Jensen, G.M., Gwyer, J., Hack, L.M., & Shepard, K.F. (2007). *Expertise in physical therapy practice* (2nd ed.). Philadelphia, PA: Saunders-Elsevier.

Jones, M.A., & Rivett, D.A. (Eds.). (2004). *Clinical reasoning for manual therapists.* Edinburgh, Scotland: Butterworth Heinemann.

Julien, H., & Boon, S. (2004). Assessing instructional outcomes in Canadian academic libraries. *Library and Information Science Research, 26*, 121–139. http://dx.doi.org/10.1016/j.lisr.2004.01.008

Katz, J. (1992). The consent principle of the Nuremberg code: Its significance then and now. In George J. Annas and Michael A. Grodin (Eds.), *The Nazi doctors and the Nuremberg code: Human rights in human experimentation* (pp. 227–239). New York: Oxford University Press.

Kloda, L.A., & Bartlett, J.C. (2014). A characterization of clinical questions asked by rehabilitation therapists. *Journal of the Medical Library Association, 102*(2), 69–77. http://dx.doi.org/10.3163/1536-5050.102.2.002

Koch, T. (1994). Establishing rigour in qualitative research: The decision trail. *Journal of Advanced Nursing, 19,* 976 – 986.

Kothari, A., Rudman, D., Dobbins, M., Rouse, M., Sibbald, S., & Edwards, N. (2012). The use of tacit and explicit knowledge in public health: A qualitative study. *Implementation Science, 7,* 20. http://dx.doi.org/10.1186/1748-5908-7-20

Kramer, B.M.R. (2010). Information retrieval: Literature searching in today's information landscape. *Hypothesis, 8*(1), 1–7. http://dx.doi.org/10.5779/hypothesis.v8i1.182

Kreitzer, M. J., Sierpina, V., & Fleishman, S. (2010). Teaching research literacy: A model faculty development program at Oregon college of oriental medicine. *Explore: The Journal of Science and Healing, 6,* 112–114. http://dx.doi.org/10.1016/j.explore.2009.12.010

Krugman, P.R. (2003). *The great unraveling: Losing our way in the new century.* New York, NY: W.W. Norton.

Lee, P. (2006). Understanding and critiquing qualitative research papers. *Nursing Times, 102*(29), 30–32.

Lee, T.-Y., Landy, C.K., Wahoush, O., Khanlou, N., Liu, Y.-C., & Li, C.-C. (2014). A descriptive phenomenology study of newcomers' experience of maternity care services: Chinese women's perspectives. *BMC Health Services Research, 14,* 114. http://dx.doi.org/10.1186/1472-6963 -14-114

Library and Archives Canada. (2016). *Welcome to the theses Canada portal.* Retrieved August 11, 2016, from www.bac-lac.gc.ca/eng/services/theses/Pages/theses-canada.aspx

Lincoln, Y.S., & Guba, E.G. (1985). *Naturalistic inquiry.* Beverly Hills, CA: Sage.

Locke, L.F., Silverman, S.J., & Spirduso, W.W. (2010). *Reading and understanding research* (3rd ed.). London, UK: Sage.

Maidment, J., Chilvers, D., Crichton-Hill, Y., & Meadows-Taurua, K. (2011). Promoting research literacy during the social work practicum. *Aotearoa New Zealand Social Work, 23*(4), 3–13. http://dx.doi.org/10.11157/anzswj-vol23iss4id145

Melnyk, B.M., & Fineout-Overholt, E. (2015). *Evidence-based practice in nursing & healthcare: A guide to best practice* (3rd ed.). Philadelphia, PA: Wolters Kluwer.

Mendeley. (2016). Mendeley [Referencing software] (Version 1). Retrieved from www.mendeley. com

Milgram, S. (1963). Behavioral study of obedience. *Journal of Abnormal and Social Psychology 67,* 371–378. Doi: 10.1037/h0040525

Modern Language Association. (2016). *MLA handbook* (8th ed.). New York, NY: Author.

Morris, Z.S., Wooding, S., & Grant, J. (2011). The answer is 17 years, what is the question: Understanding time lags in translational research. *Journal of the Royal Society of Medicine, 104,* 510–520. http://dx.doi.org/10.1258/jrsm.2011.110180

National Collaborating Centre for Methods and Tools. (2011). *Critically appraising practice guidelines: The AGREE II instrument* (Updated 1 November, 2013). Retrieved from www.nccmt.ca/resources/search/100

National Collaborating Centre for Methods and Tools. (2016). *Evidence-informed public health.* Retrieved August 11, 2016, from www.nccmt.ca/eiph/index-eng.html

National Research Council. (2012). *Using science as evidence in public policy.* Committee on the Use of Social Science Knowledge in Public Policy, K. Prewitt, T.A. Schwandt, and M.L. Straf (Eds.). Division of Behavioral and Social Sciences and Education. Washington, DC: The National Academies Press.

National Research Council Purdue University, The Writing Lab. (2016). *The Purdue online writing lab* (OWL). Retrieved August 11, 2016, from https://owl.english.purdue.edu/

Nelson, L.K. (2013). *Research in communication sciences and disorders: Methods for systematic inquiry* (2nd ed.). San Diego, CA: Plural.

Niemeijer, A.R., Depla, M.F.I.A., Frederiks, B.J.M., & Hertogh, C.M.P.M. (2015). The experiences of people with dementia and intellectual disabilities with surveillance technologies in residential care. *Nursing Ethics, 22*(3), 307–320. http://dx.doi.org/10.1177/0969733014533237

Nolan, M., & Behi, R. (1996). From methodology to method: The building blocks of research literacy. *British Journal of Nursing, 5,* 54–57. http://dx.doi.org/10.12968/bjon.1996.5.1.54

Oxman, A.D., Thomson, M.A., Davis, D.A., & Haynes, R.B. (1995). No magic bullets: A systematic review of 102 trials of interventions to improve professional practice. *Canadian Medical Association Journal, 153*, 1423–1431.

Patton, P.Q. (2015). *Qualitative research & evaluation methods* (4th ed.). Los Angeles, CA: Sage.

Pearce, M.S., Salotti, J.A., Little, M.P., McHugh, K., Lee, C., Kim, K.P., Howe, N.L., ... Berrington de Gonzalez, A. (2012). Radiation exposure from CT scans in childhood and subsequent risk of leukaemia and brain tumours: A retrospective cohort study. *Lancet, 380*(9840): 499–505.

Polanyi, M. (1968). *The tacit dimension.* New York, NY: Anchor Books.

Polanyi, M. (1998). *Personal knowledge: Towards a post-critical philosophy.* London, UK: Routledge.

Polit, D.F., & Beck, C.T. (2017). *Nursing research: Generating and assessing evidence for nursing practice* (10th ed.). Philadelphia, PA: Wolters Kluwer.

ProQuest. (n.d.). *ProQuest dissertations & theses global.* Retrieved August 11, 2016, from www.proquest.com/products-services/pqdtglobal.html

Registered Nurses' Association of Ontario. (2012). *Toolkit: Implementation of best practice guidelines* (2nd ed.). Retrieved from www.nursinglibrary.org/vhl/bitstream/10755/347395/6/RNAO_ToolKit_2012_rev4_FA.pdf

Retraction–Ileal-lymphoid-nodular hyperplasia, non-specific colitis, and pervasive developmental disorder in children. *The Lancet, 375*, 445. http://dx.doi.org/10.1016/S0140-6736(10)60175-4

Richardson, W.S., Wilson, M.C., Nishikawa, J., & Hayward, R.S. (1995). The well-built clinical question: A key to evidence-based decisions. *ACP Journal Club, 23*(3), A12–A13. http://dx.doi.org/10.7326/ACPJC-1995-123-3-A12

Roberts, M.C., & Ilardi, S.S. (2003). *Handbook of research methods in clinical psychology.* Malden, MA: Blackwell.

Rolfe, G. (2006). Validity, trustworthiness and rigour: Quality and the idea of qualitative research. *Journal of Advanced Nursing, 53*, 304–310. http://dx.doi.org/10.1111/j.1365-2648.2006.03727.x

Rycroft-Malone, J., Seers, K., Titchen, A., Harvey, G., Kitson, A., & McCormack, B. (2004). What counts as evidence in evidence-based practice? *Journal of Advanced Nursing, 47*, 81–90. http://dx.doi.org/:10.1111/j.1365-2648.2004.03068.x

Sackett, D.L., Strauss, S.E., Richardson, W.S., Rosenberg, W., & Haynes, R.B. (2000). *Evidence based medicine: How to practice and teach EBM* (2nd ed.). Edinburgh, Scotland: Churchill Livingstone.

Sandelowski, M. (1986). The problem of rigor in qualitative research. *Advances in Nursing Science, 8*(3), 27–37.

Shtarkshall, Q. (2004). *Qualitative research and evaluation methods.* Thousand Oaks, CA: Sage.

Spears, D. (2013). *Developing critical reading skills.* Dubuque, IA: McGraw-Hill.

Springett, K., & Campbell, J. (2006, November). An introductory guide to putting research into practice. Defining the research question. *Podiatry Now, 26–28.*

Straus, S.E., Tetroe, J., & Graham, I.D. (Eds.). (2009). *Knowledge translation in health care: Moving from evidence to practice.* Chichester, UK: Wiley-Blackwell.

Straus, S.E., Tetroe, J., Graham, I.D., Zwarenstein, M., & Bhattacharyya, O. (2009). Monitoring and evaluating knowledge. In: S. Straus, J. Tetroe, & I. D. Graham (Eds.), *Knowledge translation in health care* (pp. 151–159). Oxford, UK: Wiley-Blackwell.

Streubert, H.J., & Carpenter, D.R. (2011). *Qualitative research in nursing* (5th ed.). Philadelphia, PA: Wolters Kluwer.

Szumilas, M. (2010). Explaining odds ratios. *Journal of the Canadian Academy of Child and Adolescent Psychiatry, 19*, 227–229.

Tashakkori, A., & Teddlie, C. (Eds.). (2010). *SAGE handbook of mixed methods in social & behavioral research.* Thousand Oaks, CA: Sage.

Thomas, L.H., McColl, E., Cullum, N., Rousseau, N., & Soutter, J. (1999). Clinical guidelines in nursing, midwifery and the therapies: A systematic review. *Journal of Advanced Nursing, 30*, 40–50. http://dx.doi.org/10.1046/j.1365-2648.1999.01047.x

Thomas, M., Burt, M., & Parkes, J. (2010). The emergence of evidence-based practice. In J. McCarthy & P. Rose (Eds.), *Values-based health and social care beyond evidence-based practice.* London, UK: Sage.

Thomson Reuters. (2016). *Web of science*™. Retrieved August 11, 2016, from www.webofknowledge.com

Thorne, S. (2016). *Interpretive description: Qualitative research for applied practice* (2nd ed.). New York, NY: Routledge Taylor & Francis Group.

Trip Database. (2016). *Trip: Turning research into practice.* Retrieved August 11, 2016, from www.tripdatabase.com/

Trochim, W.M. (2006). *Research methods knowledge base.* Retrieved August 11, 2016, from www.socialresearchmethods.net/kb/intreval.htm

Trochim, W.M. (2016). *Qualitative vs. quantitative.* Retrieved August 11, 2016, from http://academics.lmu.edu/irb/qualitativeresearchandapproaches/qualitativevsquantitative/

United States National Library of Medicine. (2016). *Fact sheet: MEDLINE, PubMed, and PMC (PubMed Central): How are they different?* Retrieved from www.nlm.nih.gov/pubs/factsheets/dif_med_pub.html

University of Chicago. (2010). *The Chicago manual of style* (16th ed.). Retrieved from www.chicagomanualofstyle.org/tools_citationguide.html

University of York. (2015). *Centre for Reviews and Dissemination.* Retrieved at www.york.ac.uk/crd/

Wakefield, A. (2014). Searching and critiquing literature. *Nursing Standard, 28*(39), 49–57. http://dx.doi.org/10.7748/ns.28.39.49.e8867

Wakefield, A. (2015). Synthesizing the literature as part of a literature review. *Nursing Standard, 29*, 44–51. http://dx.doi.org/10.7748/ns.29.29.44.e8957

Wakefield, A., Murch, S.H., Anthony, A., Linnell, J., Casson, D.M., Malik, M., ... Walker-Smith, J.A. (1998). Ileal-lymphoid-nodular hyperplasia, non-specific colitis, and pervasive developmental disorder in children. *The Lancet, 351*, 637–641. (Retraction published in 2010, *The Lancet, 375*, 445. http://dx.doi.org/10.1016/S0140-6736(10)60175-4)

Waller, J., Bower, K.M., Spence, M., & Kavanagh, K.F. (2015). Using grounded theory methodology to conceptualize the mother-infant communication dynamic: Potential application to compliance with infant feeding recommendations. *Maternal and Child Nutrition, 11*, 749–760. http://dx.doi.org/10.1111/mcn.12056

Wayne, P.M., Buring, J.E., Davis, R.B., Andrews, S.M., John, M.S., Kerr, C.E., ... Schachter, S.C. (2008). Increasing research capacity at the New England school of acupuncture through faculty and student research training initiatives. *Alternative Therapies in Health and Medicine, 14*(2), 52–58.

Wensing, M., van der Weijden, T., & Grol, R. (1998). Implementing guidelines and innovations in general practice: Which interventions are effective? *The British Journal of General Practice, 48*, 991–997.

Williams, M.V. (2002). Recognizing and overcoming inadequate health literacy, a barrier to care. *Cleveland Clinic Journal of Medicine, 69,* 415–418. http://dx.doi.org/10.3949/ccjm.69.5.415

Williamson, G.R. (2007). *Making sense of research: An introduction for health and social care practitioners* (3rd ed.). Hoboken, NJ: Blackwell.

Wilson, K.M., Brady, T.J., & Lesesne, C. (2011). An organizing framework for translation in public health: The knowledge to action framework. *Preventing Chronic Disease, 8*(2), A46.

Woolf, S.H., Grol, R., Hutchinson, A., Eccles, M., & Grimshaw, J. (1999). Potential benefits, limitations, and harms of clinical guidelines. *BMJ, 318,* 527–530. http://dx.doi.org/10.1136/bmj.318.7182.527

World Health Organization. (2003). *Guidelines for WHO guidelines* (EIP/GPE/EQC/2003.1). Retrieved from http://apps.who.int/iris/bitstream/10665/68925/1/EIP_GPE_EQC_2003_1.pdf

World Health Organization. (2016). *Ethics and health: Ethical standards and procedures for research with human beings.* Retrieved from http://www.who.int/ethics/research/en/

Zimmer, L. (2006). Qualitative meta-synthesis: A question of dialoguing with texts. *Journal of Advanced Nursing, 53*(3), 311–318. http://dx.doi.org/10.1111/j.1365-2648.2006.03721.x